Communications in Computer and Information Science

2327

Series Editors

Gang Li ⓘ, *School of Information Technology, Deakin University, Burwood, VIC, Australia*

Joaquim Filipe ⓘ, *Polytechnic Institute of Setúbal, Setúbal, Portugal*

Zhiwei Xu, *Chinese Academy of Sciences, Beijing, China*

Rationale

The CCIS series is devoted to the publication of proceedings of computer science conferences. Its aim is to efficiently disseminate original research results in informatics in printed and electronic form. While the focus is on publication of peer-reviewed full papers presenting mature work, inclusion of reviewed short papers reporting on work in progress is welcome, too. Besides globally relevant meetings with internationally representative program committees guaranteeing a strict peer-reviewing and paper selection process, conferences run by societies or of high regional or national relevance are also considered for publication.

Topics

The topical scope of CCIS spans the entire spectrum of informatics ranging from foundational topics in the theory of computing to information and communications science and technology and a broad variety of interdisciplinary application fields.

Information for Volume Editors and Authors

Publication in CCIS is free of charge. No royalties are paid, however, we offer registered conference participants temporary free access to the online version of the conference proceedings on SpringerLink (http://link.springer.com) by means of an http referrer from the conference website and/or a number of complimentary printed copies, as specified in the official acceptance email of the event.

CCIS proceedings can be published in time for distribution at conferences or as post-proceedings, and delivered in the form of printed books and/or electronically as USBs and/or e-content licenses for accessing proceedings at SpringerLink. Furthermore, CCIS proceedings are included in the CCIS electronic book series hosted in the SpringerLink digital library at http://link.springer.com/bookseries/7899. Conferences publishing in CCIS are allowed to use Online Conference Service (OCS) for managing the whole proceedings lifecycle (from submission and reviewing to preparing for publication) free of charge.

Publication process

The language of publication is exclusively English. Authors publishing in CCIS have to sign the Springer CCIS copyright transfer form, however, they are free to use their material published in CCIS for substantially changed, more elaborate subsequent publications elsewhere. For the preparation of the camera-ready papers/files, authors have to strictly adhere to the Springer CCIS Authors' Instructions and are strongly encouraged to use the CCIS LaTeX style files or templates.

Abstracting/Indexing

CCIS is abstracted/indexed in DBLP, Google Scholar, EI-Compendex, Mathematical Reviews, SCImago, Scopus. CCIS volumes are also submitted for the inclusion in ISI Proceedings.

How to start

To start the evaluation of your proposal for inclusion in the CCIS series, please send an e-mail to ccis@springer.com.

Shalini Mahato · Bam Bahadur Sinha ·
Jayadeep Pati · Joel Rodrigues
Editors

Global Mental Health and Public Health Challenges and Innovation

First International Conference, GMHPHCI 2022
Jharkhand, India, November 25–27, 2022
Proceedings

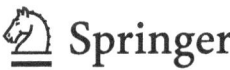

Editors
Shalini Mahato ⓘ
National Institute of Foundry and Forge
Technology (NIFFT)
Ranchi, Jharkhand, India

Jayadeep Pati ⓘ
Indian Institute of Information Technology
(IIIT)
Ranchi, Jharkhand, India

Bam Bahadur Sinha ⓘ
National Institute of Technology (NIT)
Ravangla, Sikkim, India

Joel Rodrigues ⓘ
Federal University of Piauí (UFPI)
Teresina, Brazil

ISSN 1865-0929   ISSN 1865-0937 (electronic)
Communications in Computer and Information Science
ISBN 978-3-031-82602-3   ISBN 978-3-031-82603-0 (eBook)
https://doi.org/10.1007/978-3-031-82603-0

© The Editor(s) (if applicable) and The Author(s), under exclusive license
to Springer Nature Switzerland AG 2025

This work is subject to copyright. All rights are solely and exclusively licensed by the Publisher, whether the whole or part of the material is concerned, specifically the rights of translation, reprinting, reuse of illustrations, recitation, broadcasting, reproduction on microfilms or in any other physical way, and transmission or information storage and retrieval, electronic adaptation, computer software, or by similar or dissimilar methodology now known or hereafter developed.
The use of general descriptive names, registered names, trademarks, service marks, etc. in this publication does not imply, even in the absence of a specific statement, that such names are exempt from the relevant protective laws and regulations and therefore free for general use.
The publisher, the authors and the editors are safe to assume that the advice and information in this book are believed to be true and accurate at the date of publication. Neither the publisher nor the authors or the editors give a warranty, expressed or implied, with respect to the material contained herein or for any errors or omissions that may have been made. The publisher remains neutral with regard to jurisdictional claims in published maps and institutional affiliations.

This Springer imprint is published by the registered company Springer Nature Switzerland AG
The registered company address is: Gewerbestrasse 11, 6330 Cham, Switzerland

If disposing of this product, please recycle the paper.

Dedication

This book is dedicated to all the scholars and practitioners who relentlessly pursue knowledge, fairness, and innovation. May this collection of ideas serve as a beacon for future generations.

Foreword

As we progress further into the 21st century, the importance of mental health awareness, effective treatments, and innovative public health strategies continues to grow. In this context, the International Conference on Global Mental Health and Public Health Challenges & Innovation (GMHPHCI 2022), held by the Indian Institute of Information Technology (IIIT) Ranchi, India, represents a significant endeavour to address and find solutions to these pressing issues. The conference brought together a dynamic group of scholars, practitioners, and innovators across fields, contributing invaluable insights to the global discourse on healthcare.

The proceedings of GMHPHCI-2022 reflect a pioneering effort in applying cutting-edge technologies, such as the Internet of Things (IoT), Artificial Intelligence (AI), Machine Learning (ML), and Deep Learning (DL), to tackle public and mental health challenges. These proceedings not only document the strides being made in these domains but also provide a repository of innovative ideas and solutions aimed at addressing complex healthcare issues. The conference's hybrid format enabled a wider reach, fostering a rich exchange of knowledge among international experts and inspiring cross-disciplinary collaborations that aim to reshape the landscape of mental and public health care.

This volume includes the best papers from GMHPHCI-2022, each selected through a rigorous peer-review process to ensure quality and relevance. The authors and contributors share a common vision: to advance health equity and enhance the well-being of individuals and communities worldwide. We extend our gratitude to the organizing committee, technical program committee, reviewers, and participants whose dedication and expertise have made this collection possible.

As the editors, we believe that these proceedings will inspire new approaches, foster ongoing research, and contribute to impactful healthcare policies and practices. We hope this book serves as a valuable resource for researchers, practitioners, and academicians.

Shalini Mahato
Bam Bahadur Sinha
Joel Rodrigues
Jayadeep Pati

Preface

The International Conference on Global Mental Health and Public Health Challenges and Innovation (GMHPHCI 2022) was held on 25–27th November, 2022 organized by Indian Institute of Information Technology (IIIT) Ranchi, Jharkhand, India. The conference was held in hybrid mode.

Mental health issues negatively impact millions of people globally. Mental health is an important issue with many challenges in investigation, diagnosis, treatment, monitoring, drug of choice, and side effects. Public health is the science and art of preventing disease, prolonging life, and promoting health through organized efforts and informed choices of society, organizations, public and private, communities, and individuals. Modern technologies like the Internet of Things (IoT), Artificial Intelligence (AI), Machine Learning (ML), and Deep Learning (DL), among others, could help to solve problems in the domains of mental health and public health.

GMHPHCI 2022 aimed to bring together researchers, leading scientists, psychiatrists, psychologists, doctors, statisticians, and healthcare workers to share knowledge, present their novel ideas, and discuss challenges and present novel solutions in the field of healthcare.

The conference attracted a good number of high-quality papers in the field of innovation in mental health, healthcare, and public health. A total 62 research papers were received through EasyChair and 30 papers (50%) were accepted after the rigorous review process. Seven (11.29%) papers were selected for publication in the Communications in Computer and Information Science (CCIS) series of Springer.

We extend our heartfelt gratitude to all participants of the conference. We would like to thank the entire team of GMHPHCI 2022 for their relentless effort and hard work to make the conference successful. We would like to thank the authors for submitting their papers to GMHPHCI 2022.

We are thankful to our international team of established members of the Technical Program Committee, reviewers, and everyone who was part of the conference GMHPHCI 2022.

December 2022

Shalini Mahato
Bam Bahadur Sinha
Jayadeep Pati
Joel Rodrigues

Acknowledgement

We extend our sincere gratitude to **Prof. Vishnu Priye**, Founder Director, Indian Institute of Information Technology Ranchi, for his visionary leadership and unwavering support in making the International Conference on Global Mental Health and Public Health Challenges & Innovation (GMHPHCI 2022) a remarkable success. His commitment to advancing knowledge and fostering a collaborative environment has been instrumental in bringing together scholars, practitioners, and innovators from across the globe to address pressing health issues.

We are thankful to all our authors for their valuable contribution and to the entire technical program committee team and reviewers for their support.

This commitment to interdisciplinary exchange and innovation reflects IIIT Ranchi's dedication to impacting global health positively.

We are grateful for the opportunity to host such a transformative event and look forward to many more collaborations that drive meaningful change in public and mental healthcare with future series of GMHPHCI conference.

Organization

Patron

Vishnu Priye — Indian Institute of Information Technology Ranchi, India

Convenor

Jayadeep Pati — Indian Institute of Information Technology Ranchi, India

Co-convenor

Shalini Mahato — National Institute of Advanced Manufacturing Technology, India
Bam Bahadur Sinha — National Institute of Technology Sikkim, India

Technical Program Committee

Abhishek Verma — Indian Institute of Information Technology, Design & Manufacturing Jabalpur, India
Alongbar Wary — VIT-AP University, India
Arambam Neelima — National Institute of Technology Nagaland, India
Basudeb Das — Central Institute of Psychiatry Ranchi, India
Hesam Akbari — Arizona State University, USA
Hima Bindu Kommanti — National Institute of Technology Andhra Pradesh, India
J. Arul Valan — National Institute of Technology Nagaland, India
K. G. Smitha — Nanyang Technological University, Singapore.
Karthick Sheshadri — National Institute of Technology Andhra Pradesh, India
Mahesh R. Panicker — Indian Institute of Technology Palakkad, India
Malik Yousef — Zefat Academic College, Israel
Manjunath K. V. — Indian Institute of Information Technology Dharwad, India

Nishant Goyal	Central Institute of Psychiatry Ranchi, India
Prabhu Prasad B. M.	Indian Institute of Information Technology Dharwad, India
Pramod Mane	Indian Institute of Information Technology Dharwad, India
Priyanka Sadhu	Amazon Web Services, USA
Rakesh Kumar Sinha	Birla Institute of Technology Mesra, India
S. K. Mandal	Indian Institute of Information Technology Ranchi, India
Sachi Nandan Mohanty	Singidunum University, Serbia
Sanjay Kumar Munda	Central Institute of Psychiatry Ranchi, India
Smith K. Khare	Syddansk Universitet, Denmark
Sourav Khanra	Central Institute of Psychiatry Ranchi, India
Sunil Kumar	Katholieke Universiteit Leuven, Belgium
Surendiran B.	National Institute of Technology Pondicherry, India
Tarini Mandal	Indian Institute of Information Technology Ranchi, India
Vandana	Indian Institute of Management Sirmaur, India
Varun Bajaj	Indian Institute of Information Technology Design & Manufacturing Jabalpur, India

Additional Reviewers

Aditi Sharma	Amity University Jharkhand, India
Alisha Arora	Central Institute of Psychiatry Ranchi, India
Anurag Sinha	ICFAI University, Jharkhand, India
Bhawani Sankar Panigrahi	Vardhaman College of Engineering, India
Christopher Mathew	DMMC Medical College Hospital, India
Kirti Kumari	Indian Institute of Information Technology Ranchi, India
Liza Daniel	Central Institute of Psychiatry Ranchi, India
Mallikarjunaswamy M. S.	Sri Jayachamarajendra College of Engineering, JSS Science & Technology University Mysuru, India
Manorama	Amity University Jharkhand, India
Mohammad Ahsan	University of Technology Sydney, Australia
Monika Kumari	KIIT University, India
Monika Srivastava	Indian Institute of Technology Bhilai, India
Nandini Kumari	Amity University Jharkhand, India
Neha Tigga	National Institute of Technology Jamshedpur, India

Nidhi Kushwaha	Indian Institute of Information Technology Ranchi, India
Pranjit Das	Koneru Lakshmaiah Education Foundation (Deemed to be University), India
Priyank Khare	Indian Institute of Information Technology Ranchi, India
Raganna A.	Reva University, India
Santosh Satapathy	Pandit Deendayal Energy University, India
Sravanth Kumar	University of Technology Sydney, Australia
Vani Hiremani	Symbiosis Institute of Technology Pune, India

Editorial Board

Shalini Mahato	National Institute of Advanced Manufacturing Technology, India
Bam Bahadur Sinha	National Institute of Technology Sikkim, India
Jayadeep Pati	Indian Institute of Information Technology Ranchi, India
Joel Rodrigues	Amazonas State University, Brazil

Contents

Machine Learning and Bioinformatics Analysis Reveal *POPDC3*, *FRMD5*, *CCNA1*, and *ALG1L2* as Novel Prognostic Biomarkers in Cholangiocarcinoma 1
    Aakansha Singh and Anjana Dwivedi

Automatic Detection of COVID-19 in Chest X-ray Based on VIT 12
    Kevisino Khate and Arambam Neelima

Performance Analysis of Classification and Boosting Algorithm for Diabetes Prediction 21
    Shekharesh Barik, Chandan Kumar Behera, Pravat Kumar Behera, and Subhranshu Nanda Brahmachary

An ISDUMD Algorithm Using Bayesian Averaging for Smoothing 3D Reconstruction of 2D MRI Medical Images 33
    Mriganka Sarmah, Arambam Neelima, and Puspakshi Sarmah

Traumatic Condition Assessment and Monitoring Through Retinal Fundus Image 45
    Gaurav Sharma, Maninder Singh, Basant Kumar, K. M. Soni, and Deepak Agrawal

A 1D-Convolutional Neural Network Framework with Multi-Modal Techniques for Sleep Staging System Using EEG and EOG Signals 59
    Santosh Kumar Satapathy, Hari Kishan Kondaveeti, and Vaishvi R. Shah

Review on Mental Healthcare System Using Data Analytics and IoT 72
    Mrinmoy Kayal, Mohinikanta Sahoo, and Jayadeep Pati

Author Index 79

Contributors

Deepak Agrawal All India Institute of Medical Sciences, JPNATC, New Delhi, India

Shekharesh Barik Department of CSE, DRIEMS (Autonomous), Cuttack, Odisha, India

Chandan Kumar Behera Department of CSE, DRIEMS (Autonomous), Cuttack, Odisha, India

Pravat Kumar Behera Department of CSE, DRIEMS (Autonomous), Cuttack, Odisha, India

Subhranshu Nanda Brahmachary Department of CSE, DRIEMS (Autonomous), Cuttack, Odisha, India

Anjana Dwivedi Department of Bioengineering and Biotechnology, Birla Institute of Technology, Mesra, Jharkhand, India

Mrinmoy Kayal Department of Computer Science and Engineering, Indian Institute of Information Technology Ranchi, Ranchi, Jharkhand, India

Kevisino Khate Department of Computer Science and Engineering, National Institute of Technology, Chumukedima, Nagaland, India

Hari Kishan Kondaveeti School of Computer Science Engineering, VIT-AP University, Vijayawada, Andhra Pradesh, India

Basant Kumar Electronics and Communication Engineering Department, Motilal Nehru National Institute of Technology Allahabad, Prayagraj, India

Arambam Neelima Department of Computer Science and Engineering, National Institute of Technology, Chumukedima, Nagaland, India

Arambam Neelima CSE, NIT, Dimapur, Nagaland, India

Jayadeep Pati Department of Computer Science and Engineering, Indian Institute of Information Technology Ranchi, Ranchi, Jharkhand, India

Mohinikanta Sahoo Department of Computer Science and Engineering, Indian Institute of Information Technology Ranchi, Ranchi, Jharkhand, India

Mriganka Sarmah CSE, NIT, Dimapur, Nagaland, India

Puspakshi Sarmah CS, NEF College, Guwahati, Assam, India

Santosh Kumar Satapathy Information and Communication Technology, Pandit Deendayal Energy University, Gandhinagar, Gujarat, India

Vaishvi R. Shah Information and Communication Technology, Pandit Deendayal Energy University, Gandhinagar, Gujarat, India

Gaurav Sharma Amity Institute of Information Technology, Amity University, Noida, India

Aakansha Singh Department of Bioengineering and Biotechnology, Birla Institute of Technology, Mesra, Jharkhand, India

Maninder Singh Electronics and Communication Engineering Department, Motilal Nehru National Institute of Technology Allahabad, Prayagraj, India

K. M. Soni Amity Institute of Information Technology, Amity University, Noida, India

List of Abbreviation

AHI	Apnea-Hypopnea Index
ABP	Arterial Blood Pressure
AI	Artificial Intelligence
BAM	Bayesian Averaging Method
BELM	Bayesian Extreme Learning Machines
BR	Bayesian Regulation
BESO	Bi-directional ESO
BPD	Borderline Personality Disorder
CBF	Cerebral Blood Flow
CPP	Cerebral Perfusion Pressure
CSF	Cerebrospinal Fluid
CCA	Cholangiocarcinoma
CT	Computed Tomography
CLAHE	Contrast Limited Adaptive Histogram Equalization
CNN	Convolutional Neural Network
Cox PH	Cox Proportional Hazard
DL	Deep Learning
DS	Deep Sleep
DRIVE	Digital Retinal Images For Vessel Extraction
EEG	Electroencephalogram
EOG	Electromyogram
EOGs	Electrooculograms
EEMD	Ensemble Empirical Mode Decomposition
ESO	Evolutionary Structural Optimization Method
fMRI	Functional Magnetic Resonance Imaging
GLM	General Linear Model
HRCT	High-Resolution Computed Tomography
HRF	High-Resolution Fundus
HC	Humphrey's Class
IIH	Idiopathic Intracranial Hypertension
INSPIRE-AVR	Iowa Normative Set For Processing Images Of The Retina
IHR	Instantaneous Heart Rate
IoT	Internet Of Things
ICP	Intracranial Pressure
IMFs	Intrinsic Mode Functions
KNN	K-Nearest Neighbors
LSE	Least Square Error
LM	Levenberg Marquardt
LS	Light Sleep
ML	Machine Learning
MRI	Magnetic Resonance Imaging

MC	Marching Cube
MCF	Mean Curvature Flow
MSE	Mean Squared Error
MHSA	Multi-Head Self-Attention
MLP	Multi-Layer Perceptron
OSA	Obstructive Sleep Apnea
PDEs	Partial Differential Equations
PSG	Polysomnographic
PNN	Probabilistic Neural Network
PL	Product-Limit
QSSA	Quaternion-valued Singular Spectrum Analysis
REM	Rapid Eye Movement Stage
RITE	Retinal Images Vessel Tree Extraction
SDU	Scale Dependant Umbrella
SCG	Scaled Conjugate Gradient
SIMP	Solid Isotropic Material with Penalization
STARE	Structured Analysis of The Retina
SGD	Stochastic Gradient Descent
SVM	Support Vector Machine
TCGA	The Cancer Genome Atlas
CDR	Cup To Disc Ratio
VIT	Vision Transformer

Machine Learning and Bioinformatics Analysis Reveal *POPDC3, FRMD5, CCNA1,* and *ALG1L2* as Novel Prognostic Biomarkers in Cholangiocarcinoma

Aakansha Singh[✉] [iD] and Anjana Dwivedi [iD]

Department of Bioengineering and Biotechnology, Birla Institute of Technology, Mesra 835215, Jharkhand, India
{phdbe10057.20,anjana.dwivedi}@bitmesra.ac.in

Abstract. Cholangiocarcinoma (CCA) is a heterogenous malignancy that can occur anywhere along the biliary tract. Its heterogeneous and aggressive behaviour necessitates the identification of biomarkers influencing the overall survival of patients. The current work utilizes clinical and RNA-Seq data of 36 CCA patients from the TCGA database. Cox Proportional Hazard (Cox PH) model was employed to evaluate the transcriptomic information and clinical factors in determining their relative effects on patient survival. The univariate analysis revealed that FRMD5, CCNA1, ALG1L2, and POPDC3 genes are significantly related to the patient's survival, while the multivariate analysis done for all the genes together confirmed a significant relation of some genes on the overall survival. And, the combined analysis of clinical and transcriptomic data suggests that mutation counts, neoplasmic grade, and patient's weight are significantly correlated with the patient's survival. Additionally, the expression pattern of selected genes was validated using the firebrowse database. This integrated analytical study reveals *POPDC3, FRMD5, CCNA1,* and *ALG1L2* as novel and crucial prognostic biomarkers of CCA and their high expression correlates to poor survival of CCA patients.

Keywords: Machine learning · Bioinformatics · Survival analysis · Cox regression model · Cholangiocarcinoma

1 Introduction

Cholangiocarcinoma (CCA) is a highly lethal adenocarcinoma of the hepatobiliary tract comprising a cluster of heterogeneous tumors. There is a steady rise in the incidence of CCA contributing to around 15% of all liver cancers and about 3% of gastrointestinal tract cancers [1]. A majority of CCA patients reported a delayed diagnosis, rapid tumor progression, and poor survival pointing towards surgery as the only curative treatment. However, in most cases, the patients are not surgical candidates. The present 5-year survival rate of CCA patients after the surgery and chemotherapy is <20% [2] which necessitates the identification of novel biomarkers for diagnosis and therapeutics. High-throughput technologies like microarray and RNA-Seq analysis are being efficiently utilized in cancer investigation and research, generating a plethora of raw data which can be further analyzed through new knowledge-based methods *viz.* Application of computer science, artificial intelligence, machine learning, and statistics along with traditional approaches. Fortunately, these data can be integrated with bioinformatics and machine learning tools to analyze and discover new findings. Identifying new biomarkers that are associated with CCA progression and survival can be of immense importance in cancer research. The Cancer Genome Atlas (TCGA) is a repository that avails the clinical, survival, transcriptomics, mutation, methylation, and many more data of real-world cancer patients. The clinical parameters and transcriptomic data are highly useful in identifying novel biomarkers. In 2020, Wang et al. investigated the TCGA dataset using a bioinformatics and network biology-based approach and looked into the potential roles of AURKB and PLK1 in the diagnosis and prognosis of CCA patients [3]. Wang et. al. in 2022 identified three prognostic-related genes (BEST1, CCL2, and PLAUR) of CCA involved in inflammation-related response by utilizing bioinformatics and machine learning approach [4].

Despite recent advancements in clinical research, limited biomarkers are known that are associated with the diagnosis and prognosis of CCA. Therefore, in the present work, we intend to explore some crucial prognostic genes by employing Cox Proportional Hazard (Cox PH) models on clinical and transcriptomic data of CCA patients. The publicly available TCGA dataset (RNA-Seq and clinical) of 36 CCA patients was considered to identify the significant association in CCA prognosis.

2 Materials and Methodology

2.1 Data Retrieval and Processing

The CCA patients' data (Cholangiocarcinoma, TCGA, PanCancer Atlas) was retrieved through the cBioPortal platform. The clinical data consisted of 36 cases and 54 attributes while the RNA-Seq data contained 36 cases and 17734 mutated genes. To investigate the influence of genetic alterations and clinical attributes on the overall survival of patients, six clinical features (diagnosis age, sex, cancer stage, neoplasmic grade, mutation count, and aneuploidy score) (Table 1) along with 38 most altered genes was utilized. Both clinical and RNA-Seq data were matched according to the patient's ids and survival data were taken as overall survival months and status. For comparing the expression alterations between patients and control we considered the *z-score* values. The genes with z-score values $\geq +1.5$ and ≤ -1.5 are considered DEGs and any numbers in between this threshold value as normal.

2.2 Analytical Methods Used

The RNA-Seq and clinical data were merged according to the patient's barcode information and a single file was obtained for subsequent analyses. Initially, Cox PH models were employed for univariate and multivariate analysis. This model has been previously

Table 1. Clinical features selected for the analysis

Features	Category	Frequency
Diagnostic age	≤55	09
	>55	27
Mutation count	≤30	13
	>30	23
Sex	Male	16
	Female	20
Patient's Weight	≤75	18
	>75	18
Aneuploidy score	≤10	25
	>10	09
Neoplasmic grade	Grade I	01
	Grade II	15
	Grade III	18
	Grade IV	02

used for the survival analysis of several cancer patients [5] which depicts the dependency of survival time on predictor variables. The Cox model can be written as:

$$h(t) = h_0(t) \times \exp(b1_{x1} + b2_{x2} + \cdots + bp_{xp}) \quad (1)$$

Here, h(t) represents the hazard function determined by covariates p (x_1, x_2,..., x_p), t = survival time, b_1, b_2,..., b_p = coefficients that measure the impact of covariates, h_0 = baseline hazard function.

Kaplan-Meier product-limit (PL) estimator was used to analyze the survival function of patients [6] which can be calculated by:

$$S(ti) = Sx^2(ti-1)(1 - \frac{di}{ni}) \quad (2)$$

Here, $S(t_i)$ is the survival probability at time t_i, $S(t_{i-1})$ is the probability of a patient being alive at time t_{i-1}, d_i is the number of events at ti, and n_i is the number of patients alive just before the t_i. Estimation of survival function was done followed by the Log-rank test to compare the significant difference in the gene expression between the two groups. The following null and alternative hypotheses can be designed for comparing the altered and normal expression:

$$H_0 : S_{altered}(t) = S_{normal}(t) \quad (3)$$

$$H_A : S_{altered}(t) \neq S_{normal}(t) \quad (4)$$

Here, the null hypothesis (H_0) states that the survival function is the same for both altered and normal cases while the alternate hypothesis (H_A) states the survival function is not the same in altered and normal groups.

After the identification of genes exhibiting a significant difference in normal and altered groups, Cox regression analysis was done. Initially, a univariate analysis was performed for each gene separately followed by a multivariate survival analysis of all 38 genes simultaneously. Then, a Cox PH model was fitted to six clinical features and 38 genes to infer the influence of different factors on a patient's survival. This approach is useful in estimating the effect of a specific gene on the survival of patients in the presence of clinical factors [7]. Thereafter, the expression of identified genes was validated using the firebrowse database. Upon validating the expression profile of genes, further interest was to identify the different proteins that closely interact with these genes, and the PPI networks were constructed for validated genes using the STRING database and visualized through Cytoscape. Finally, the GO and KEGG pathway analysis was conducted for the prognostic genes and their interacting proteins using the DAVID tool.

3 Results

3.1 Survival Function Analysis of Altered Genes

A PL estimator analysis done to assess the relation between gene alteration and patients' survival based on a log-rank test revealed an association of some genes with overall survival. The genes were selected based on p-values. Generally, a p-value <0.05 is considered to be significant [8]. Figure 1a–d demonstrates the overall survival prediction of patients considering the gene expression. From the Figures provided, it can be seen that the survival probability of patients deteriorates if the expression of *CCA3, FRMD5, CCNA1,* and *ALG1L2* is high.

Fig. 1. (a–d): Kaplan-Meier plot showing the survival probability of patients based on the high and low expression of genes, 1a- POPDC3, 1b- FRMD5, 1c-CCNA1, and 1d- ALG1L2.

3.2 Fitting Cox PH Model with RNA-Seq and Clinical Data

The Cox regression model is a popularly used method in investigating the effect of various factors associated with overall patient survival [9]. **Univariate** and **multivariate regression models** were fitted to assess the influence of gene alterations and clinical factors on survival. Table 2, presents the result of the univariate analysis. Here, in the table, only those genes are listed that were found significant (p-value < 0.05), the rest of the genes showed some insignificant p-values. The result shows that expression of *POPDC3, FRMD5, ALG1L2,* and *CCNA1* were statistically significant and suggests that these genes are associated with the survival of CCA patients. The result of the multivariate analysis (shown in Table 3) suggests that *POPDC3, PLF5P, GDF5, GJB6,* and *FAM81B* were statistically significant concerning the overall survival. *POPDC3* was found to be common in both univariate and multivariate analysis, while the expression of *FAM81B* was significant only in multivariate analysis. Studies suggest that a hazard ratio > 1 is associated with poor survival of patients [10].

Table 2. Summary of significant genes obtained from univariate Cox PH model analysis

Genes	β	HR	p-value
CCNA1	1.439	4.217	0.014
ALG1L2	–0.636	0.529	0.049
FRMD5	1.126	3.083	0.000
POPDC3	1.851	6.365	0.007

Table 3. Summary of significant genes obtained from multivariate Cox PH model analysis

Genes	β	HR	p-value
PLK5P	2.308	10.057	0.022
POPDC3	5.295	199.433	0.003
FAM81B	4.528	92.562	0.013
GJB6	–4.358	0.013	0.008
GDF5	–4.449	0.012	0.008

The result of the combined analysis (RNA-Seq data and clinical factors) is shown in Table 4 and includes only the significant variables. From Table 4, it can be observed that the clinical features like mutation counts, age at the time of diagnosis, and patient's weight are significant and influence the overall survival of patients. Interestingly, the association between neoplasmic grade and aneuploidy score was not statistically significant with survival. And, the analysis carried out for genes showed that *POPDC3, ALG1L2, FAM81B, HIST1B, GDF5, GJB6, FRMD5,* and *PLK5P* were statistically significant. Notably, the expression of *POPDC3* was significant in all three analyses. The expression of *FAM81B, GDF5, GJB6,* and *PLK5P* was significant in multivariate and combined multivariate analysis.

The overall analysis shows that 6 genes (*FAM81B, POPDC3, PLK5P, ALG1L2, FRMD5, and CCNA1*) among the 38 genes, were involved in influencing the overall survival. However, the result in Table 2 suggests that the expression of *POPDC3, FRMD5, CCNA1,* and *ALG1L2* can independently influence the survival of CCA patients.

3.3 Gene Expression Validation of Prognostic Biomarkers

Results from previous steps predicted *POPDC3, FRMD5, CCNA1,* and *ALG1L2* to be the potential biomarkers in prognosing CCA. This was validated using the firebrowse

Table 4. Summary of results obtained from combined analysis of clinical features and RNA-Seq data

Variables	β	HR	p-value
Mutation count	0.026	0.974	0.007
Age at the time of diagnosis	0.081	1.084	0.015
Weight	0.233	1.262	0.051
CCNA1	4.264	71.083	0.024
ALG1L2	15.903	8062272.261	0.042
POPDC3	14.167	1420891.960	0.001
PLP	12.779	354541.324	0.019
FRMD5	−14.227	0.000	0.014
GDF5	−15.621	0.000	0.015
GJB6	−11.484	0.000	0.004
FAM81B	14.414	1819600.635	0.007

database to compare the gene expression. Box plots in Figs. 2a–d illustrate the expression of genes in tumor vs normal samples. The expression patterns of genes were found to be

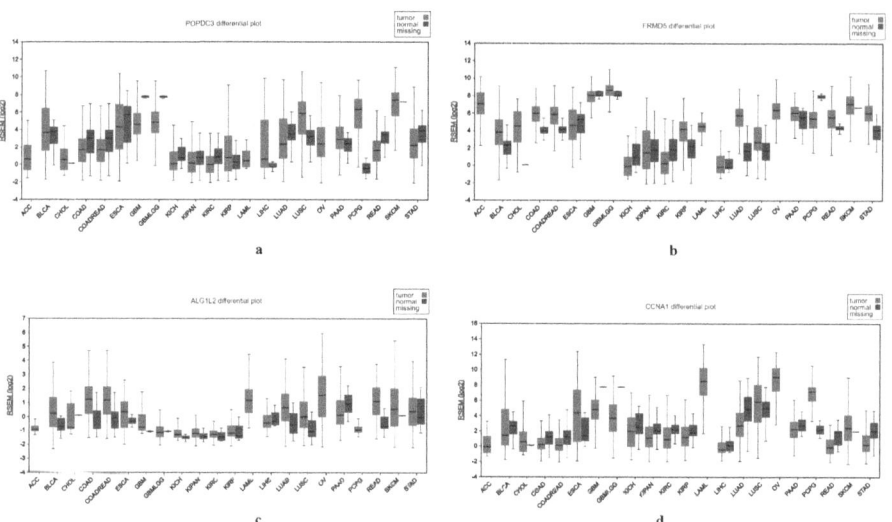

Fig. 2. (a–d): Results of gene expression profiling obtained from the firebrowse database. Box plots in red denote the gene expression in the tumor sample and the blue ones are of normal samples, while the box plots in grey denote the missing data. 2a- POPDC3, 2b- FRMD5, 2c- ALG1L2, and 2d- CCNA1. The expression of genes compared for CCA patients is highlighted with dotted lines. The above plots show a significant difference in gene expression between tumor and normal samples. (Color figure online)

comparatively higher in cancer patients, validating the results obtained from the Cox PH model analysis. Remarkably, the expression of *FRMD5* was significantly much higher than the rest of the genes.

3.4 PPI Analysis of Prognostic Genes

The network of FRMD5 consisted of 21 nodes and 60 edges with 11 proteins in direct interaction. The network of POPDC3 contained 21 nodes and 55 edges with 10 proteins in direct interaction. ALG1L2 network contained 21 nodes and 69 edges and 14 proteins

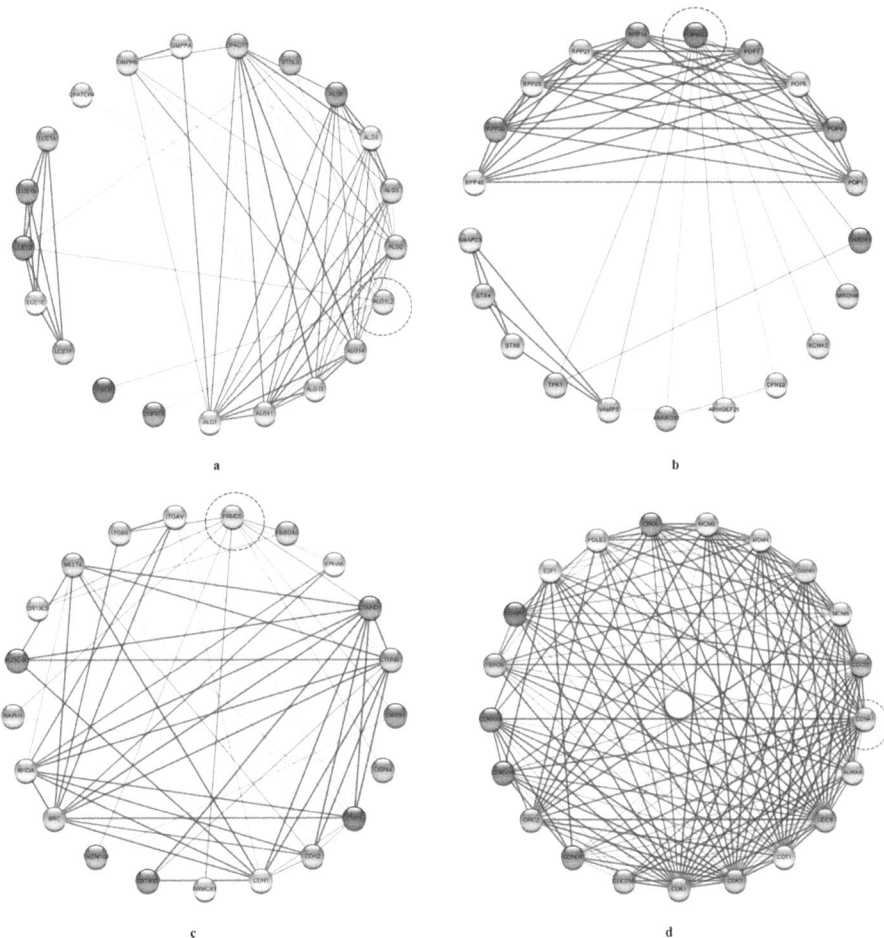

Fig. 3. (a–d): Protein interaction networks of individual prognosis-related genes identified from our analysis. 3a shows the interaction of ALG1l2 with their neighbouring proteins, 3b shows the interaction of POPDC3, 3c shows the interaction of FRMd5 and 3d shows the interaction of CCNA1 with their neighbouring proteins. These networks are constructed with a confidence score >0.4.

were directly interacting with ALG1L2, while CCNA1 consisted of 21 nodes and 165 edges with 18 proteins in direct interaction (Fig. 3a–d).

3.5 GO and KEGG Pathway Enrichment Analysis

To evaluate the involvement of identified genes and their interacting proteins in different pathways, GO and KEGG pathway analysis was done using the DAVID bioinformatics tool (Tables 4 and 5). GO analysis revealed the involvement of these genes in biological processes like a response to drugs, positive regulation of cell proliferation and migration, negative regulation of the apoptotic process, etc. Additionally, these genes were found to be involved in pathways like N-Glycan biosynthesis, bladder cancer, gastric cancer,cushing syndrome, and adherens junctions. (Table 6).

Table 5. Gene Ontology analysis of genes and their associated biological processes obtained from the DAVID database.

GO Term	Biological Process	Genes Involved	p-value
GO:0042493	response to drug	CDKN1A, CDKN1B, CCND1, CDH1, SRC, CDK1, RPP21	2.43E–05
GO:0008284	positive regulation of cell proliferation	CDC20, CDKN1B, CDK2, ITGAV, STX4, FBXO5, CDC25B	0.023851
GO:0043066	negative regulation of the apoptotic process	CDKN1A, CDKN1B, SRC, CDK1, CTNNB1, AURKA	0.022181
GO:0034446	substrate adhesion-dependent cell spreading	SRC, ITGAV, RHOA, VAMP3	0.001681
GO:0030335	positive regulation of cell migration	CDH5, ITGAV, STX4, RHOA	0.03615

4 Discussion

The present study utilizes an integrated machine learning and bioinformatics approach to elucidate the influence of gene alterations and clinical features on the overall survival of CCA patients. PL-based survival function and Cox PH models' analyses were used followed by several bioinformatics analyses to achieve a comprehensive knowledge of identified biomarkers, their biological processes, and interacting proteins.

From the analyses, some of the novel biomarkers were identified associated with the prognosis of CCA. The univariate analysis revealed four independent prognostic biomarkers *(POPDC3, FRMD5, CCNA1,* and *ALG1L2).* Five genes *(FAM81B, GJB6, GDF5, PLK5P,* and *POPDC3)* were identified from multivariate analysis and eight significant genes *(FAM81B, HIST1B, GJB6, GDF5, FRMD5, PLK5P, ALG1L2,* and *POPDC3)* were obtained from combined analysis.

Table 6. Pathway enrichment analysis of genes showing their involvement in various cancer-related pathways.

KEGG Term	Pathway Involved	Genes	p-value
hsa00510	N-Glycan biosynthesis	DPAGT1, ALG6, ALG5, ALG14, ALG2, ALG3, ALG13, ALG1, ALG11	9.34E–10
hsa05219	Bladder cancer	CDKN1A, CCND1, CDH1, SRC, E2F1	1.45E–04
hsa05226	Gastric cancer	CDKN1A, CDKN1B, CCND1, CDH1, CDK2, E2F1, CTNNB1	4.21E–04
hsa04934	Cushing syndrome	CDKN1A, CDKN1B, CCND1, CDK2, E2F1, CTNNB1, KCNK2	5.20E–04
hsa04520	Adherens junction	CDH1, SRC, CTNND1, CTNNB1, RHOA	0.001201

POPDC3 is a membrane protein-coding gene that is involved in cyclic adenosine monophosphate (cAMP) signaling. Recent studies suggest a potential role of *POPDC3* in cancer progression and prognosis. The up-regulation of POPDC3 in head and neck squamous cell carcinoma (HNSCC) patients was associated with poor survival of patients [11]. Another investigation of breast carcinoma reported the overexpression of POPDC3 in malignant tumor tissues [12]. The expression profile shown in Fig. 3a validates the results obtained from our statistical analysis. FRMD5 is a novel protein reported to be involved in cancer progression. A recent study by Zhu et.al., 2017 reports it as a novel target of the β-catenin/ TCF7L2 complex [13]. In human lung cancer cells, FRMD5 was found to regulate cell migration by interacting with integrin β and ROCK1 [14]. The accumulation of β-catenin transactivates the TCF7L2 complex which further deregulates Wnt-pathway and supports cancer progression [15]. The enhanced expression of FRMD5 in HNSCC and papillary thyroid carcinoma promotes carcinogenesis and metastasis [16, 17]. CCNA1 proteins are known to be an important cell-cycle regulator of the G1/S phase. It activates CDK1 and CDK2 and promotes cell-cycle progression [18]. The involvement of this gene is reported in the MAPK-ERK pathway and a direct association has been reported in the progression of thyroid cancer [19]. Mutations and alterations in gene expression of CCNA1 have been observed in cancers like breast carcinoma, urothelial carcinoma, and others [20]. ALG1L2 gene is involved in glycosylation. Not much information about this gene is provided in the literature. However, the copy number variation and genetic aberrations have been studied for proctitis (inflammation of the rectum) in European people. The transcriptomic profiling revealed the association of ALG1L2 with Proctitis. GO and pathway analysis revealed its role as mannosyl transferase in protein glycosylation [21]. The role of AL1G1L2 was investigated in patients with neuropathic pain and a significant difference in gene expression was found in patients with neuropathic pain when compared to individuals without pain [22]. A recent study on uveal melanoma, a most common intraocular malignancy reported a frequent genetic mutation in the ALG1L2 gene. Moreover, the role of ALG1L2 has not been explored in other cancers.

GO and KEGG pathway analysis of these genes and their interacting proteins revealed their role in various cancer-promoting pathways like positive regulation of cell proliferation, transforming growth factor beta receptor signaling pathway, positive regulation of cell migration, and many more. These pathways play a critical role in the progression of CCA and are directly related to the poor survival of patients. Among the 38 genes, we report *POPDC3, FRMD5, CCNA1,* and *ALG1L2* as prominent prognostic biomarkers of CCA influencing the overall survival of patients.

5 Conclusions

This study utilized the machine learning and bioinformatics approaches on the RNA-Seq and clinical data to unveil their influence on the overall survival of CCA patients. Among the clinical features studied, mutation count, the weight of patients, and age at the time of diagnosis, negatively correlates with the patient's survival. We report four *novel* prognostic biomarkers *(POPDC3, FRMD5, CCNA1,* and *ALG1L2)* whose upregulation is associated with poor survival of CCA patients. The role of the above-reported genes has not been yet explored in CCA making them crucial for further research and in-vitro validation. We believe that this kind of integrative analysis helps predict potential biomarkers that can be further validated *in-vitro* and *in-vivo*.

Acknowledgments. Not Applicable.

Author's Contribution. Dr. Anjana Dwivedi conceptualized this work, Experimentation and manuscript preparation were done by Aakansha Singh, and manuscript editing and the final draft was approved by Anjana Dwivedi. This work was done under the supervision of Dr. Anjana Dwivedi. The manuscript was read and approved by both the authors.

References

1. Dechêne, A., Kasper, S.: Gastroenterologe **11**(5), 400–409 (2016). https://doi.org/10.1007/s11377-016-0096-2
2. Oliveira, I.S., Kilcoyne, A., Everett, J.M., Mino-Kenudson, M., Harisinghani, M.G., Ganesan, K.: Cholangiocarcinoma: Classification, diagnosis, staging, imaging features, and management. Abdom Radiol (NY) **42**, 1637–1649 (2017)
3. Wang, K., Zhang, Y., Yang, X., Chen, T., Han, T.: Analysis of differentially expressed mRNAs and the prognosis of cholangiocarcinoma based on TCGA database. Trans. Cancer Res. **9**(8), 4739 (2020)
4. Wang, Y., Chen, S., He, S.: Bioinformatics analysis of inflammation gene signature in indicating cholangiocarcinoma prognosis. J. Oncol. (2022)
5. Amico, M., Van Keilegom, I.: Cure models in survival analysis. Ann. Rev. Stat. Appl. **5**, 311–342 (2018)
6. Deo, S.V., Deo, V., Sundaram, V.: Survival analysis—part 2: Cox proportional hazards model. Ind. J. Thoracic Cardiovascul. Surg. **37**(2), 229–233 (2021)

7. Zuo, S., Zhang, X., Wang, L.: A RNA sequencing-based six-gene signature for survival prediction in patients with glioblastoma. Sci. Rep. **9**(1), 1–10 (2019)
8. Reid, N., Cox, D.R.: Analysis of Survival Data. Chapman and Hall/CRC (2018)
9. Di Leo, G., Sardanelli, F.: Statistical significance: p value, 0.05 threshold, and applications to radiomics—reasons for a conservative approach. Euro. Radiol. Exp. **4**(1), 1–8 (2020)
10. Sashegyi, A., Ferry, D.: On the interpretation of the hazard ratio and communication of survival benefit. Oncologist **22**(4), 484–486 (2017)
11. He, X., et al.: POPDC3 is a potential biomarker for prognosis and radioresistance in patients with head and neck squamous cell carcinoma. Oncol. Lett. **18**(5), 5468–5480 (2019)
12. Amunjela, J.N., Tucker, S.J.: POPDC1 is suppressed in human breast cancer tissues and is negatively regulated by EGFR in breast cancer cell lines. Cancer Lett. **406**, 81–92 (2017)
13. Furukawa, Y., et al.: Identification of FERM domain-containing protein 5 (FRMD5) as a novel target of β-catenin/TCF7L2 complex. Cancer Res. **77**(13_Supplement), 318–318 (2017)
14. Hu, J., et al.: FERM domain-containing protein FRMD5 regulates cell motility via binding to integrin β5 subunit and ROCK1. FEBS Lett. **588**(23), 4348–4356 (2014)
15. Balza, E., Zanellato, S., Poggi, A., Reverberi, D., Rubartelli, A.: Suppressors of cytokine signaling: potential immune checkpoint molecules for cancer immunotherapy (2017)
16. Mao, X., et al.: C-terminal truncated HBx protein activates caveolin-1/LRP6/β-catenin/FRMD5 axis in promoting hepatocarcinogenesis. Cancer Lett. **444**, 60–69 (2019)
17. Gaweł, A.M., et al.: Analysis of the role of FRMD5 in the biology of papillary thyroid carcinoma. Int. J. Mol. Sci. **22**(13), 6726 (2021)
18. Sun, Q., Shi, R., Wang, X., Li, D., Wu, H., Ren, B.: Overexpression of ZIC5 promotes proliferation in non-small cell lung cancer. Biochem. Biophys. Res. Commun. **479**(3), 502–509 (2016)
19. da Silva, R.M., et al.: CCNA1 gene as a potential diagnostic marker in papillary thyroid cancer. Acta Histochemica **122**(8), 151635 (2020)
20. Munari, E., et al.: Cyclin A1 expression predicts progression in pT1 urothelial carcinoma of bladder: a tissue microarray study of 149 patients treated by transurethral resection. Histopathology **66**, 262–269 (2015)
21. Pathak, G.A., Polimanti, R., Silzer, T.K., Wendt, F.R., Chakraborty, R., Phillips, N.R.: Genetically-regulated transcriptomics & copy number variation of proctitis points to altered mitochondrial and DNA repair mechanisms in individuals of European ancestry. BMC Cancer **20**(1), 1–13 (2020)
22. Held, M., et al.: Sensory profiles and immune-related expression patterns of patients with and without neuropathic pain after peripheral nerve lesion. Pain **160**(10), 2316–2327 (2019)

Automatic Detection of COVID-19 in Chest X-ray Based on VIT

Kevisino Khate(✉) and Arambam Neelima

Department of Computer Science and Engineering, National Institute of Technology, Chumukedima 797103, Nagaland, India
kevisinokhate@nitnagaland.ac.in

Abstract. The World Health Organization reported the covid-19 virus a global pandemic on March 11, 2020. The RT-PCR test, also known as reverse polymerase chain reaction is used to determine the ailment. It does, however, suffer from false negative. Due to its potential to rapidly mutate, early discovery of the disease is essential for combating its further spread. Medical imaging approaches including Computed Tomography (CT), chest X-rays and computer vision techniques are used to assess covid-19. A vision transformer (VIT) based model for covid-19 detection in chest X-ray images is proposed. Contrast Limited Adaptive Histogram Equalization (CLAHE) and Gaussian Filter is used in the preprocessing step to improve the contrast of the chest X-rays images. The study compares the proposed technique to pre-trained convolutional neural network (CNN) models.

Keywords: Health care · covid-19 · detection · Artificial Intelligence · Image processing

1 Introduction

Coronavirus is an ailment caused by the SARS-CoV-2 virus. The World Health Organization has labelled it as a global pandemic because of its contagiousness and capacity to rapidly mutate. Spread of the infection can be stopped if it is discovered early on. Reverse Transcription Polymerase Chain Reaction is utilized for covid-19 disease diagnosis but it suffers from false negatives. Medical imaging encompasses a variety of modalities used to examine the internal organs or tissues of a person in order to identify or diagnose disease. There are many modalities of digital medical images and their uses differ according to the types of conditions it deals with. Some existing medical modalities are CT, Chest X-rays and Magnetic Resonance Imaging. A patient health can be ascertained through the use of medical images. Medical images are crucial in detecting novel coronavirus. Covid-19 can impact various organs and induce initial symptoms such as fever, flu, cardiovascular damage and pulmonary injury. Image processing, Machine Learning (ML) and Deep Learning (DL) vision transformer approach were applied to distinguish the novel coronavirus. This paper contains the following sections: The pertinent literature is presented in Sect. 2, and the proposed work is described in Sect. 3, while Sects. 4, 5 and 6 describe the analysis of the experiment, the evaluation metrics, the results and the discussion. In Sect. 7, the paper is concluded.

2 Related Work

This section discusses in depth the many approaches used to detect new coronavirus. In [1] the author employed support vector machine (SVM), Bayesian network and Random Forest algorithm. SVM achieved the best result among the three methods, making it a better choice. In [2] the author recommended using Bayesnet classifier to detect covid-19 disease on 453 covid-19 positive and 497 normal dataset samples. Ardakani et al. [3] proposed the use of KNN and SVM. In [4] the author uses Histogram of Oriented Gradient and convolutional neural network. Panwar et al. [5] developed the nCOVnet method to detect COVID-19 disease. In [6], the author has proposed XVITCOS, which is based on Vision Transformer (VIT).

2.1 Transfer Learning

Transfer learning is a common deep learning approach in which information obtained during model training on enormous datasets is transferred to some other model targeted at handling a task similar to the original task. VGGNet, Inception V3, ResNet, Xception, and MobileNet [7] are few of the well known state of the art (SOTA) pre-trained models trained on the ImageNet dataset. Narin et al. [8] suggested using InceptionV3 and Inception-ResNetv2, ResNet50, ResNet101, ResNet152 to determine the disease. In [9], Deep transfer learning methods such as ResNet, SqueezeNet, and DenseNet121 were used to identify covid-19.

2.2 Inception V3

Inception [10] is a classification network built on CNN. It is 48 layers deep and employs inception modules, each of which consists of a concatenation layer with 1×1, 3×3 and 5×5. GoogleNet is another name for this network. One of the most import aspects of an inception network is the fact that it runs a number of convolution layers in parallel at the same time. The classification layer is linked up with the average pooling layer in a straightforward manner without going via the fully connected layer.

2.3 MobileNet

MobileNet [11] is an architecture that makes use of depthwise separable convolutions to build lightweight deep convolutional neural networks. The model was created for usage in computer applications. A depthwise seperable convolution consists of two processes, which are referred to as the pointwise convolution and the depthwise convolution, respectively. While the pointwise convolution filter linearly combines the depthwise convolution output with 1×1 convolutions, the depthwise convolution filter is used to give each input channel a single convolution.

3 Materials and Methods

Many of the articles mentioned above have class imbalance and image noise issues. In order to circumvent these drawbacks, the aforementioned research uses a wide variety of image preprocessing techniques namely Contrast Limited Adaptive Histogram Equalization (CLAHE) and Gaussian filter. Furthermore, a fine-tuned vision transformer (VIT) based model [12] is used to improve covid-19 identification accuracy. The finetuned model is depicted in a schematic format in Fig. 1. Then, a comparison is done between this model and the pre-trained CNN.

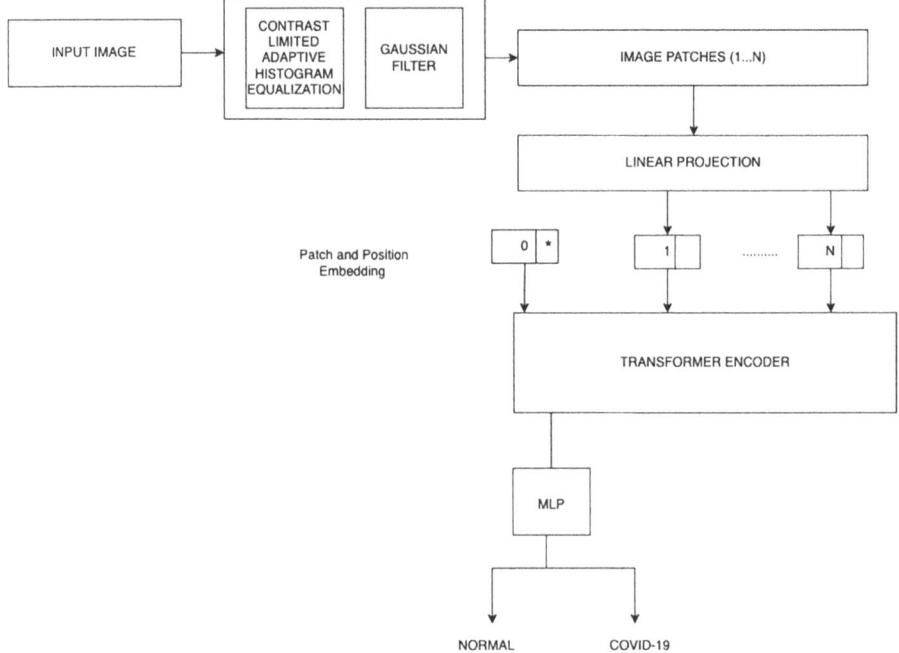

Fig. 1. Block diagram of the finetuned model

3.1 Dataset

In order to evaluate the efficiency of the proposed method, COVID-19 Radiography Database [13] are used. This dataset was compiled by a community of researchers [14] and medical experts. Utilizing 3617 covid-19 and 3617 normal chest X-ray images, the proposed approach is evaluated.

3.2 Image Pre-processing

Image enhancement is a technique used to improve the image quality. It incorporates both spatial and frequency domain techniques. The input chest X-ray images are resized to 224 × 224 in the preprocessing stage, and then CLAHE and Gaussian filter are used to minimize noise.

3.2.1 Contrast Limited Adaptive Histogram Equalization (CLAHE)

A graphical representation of the intensity distribution of an image is called a histogram. When the histogram of an image is restricted to a limited area, histogram equalization is effective. It will not perform effectively in regions where there are significant changes in intensity and when the histogram covers a large area. Adaptive Histogram Equalization (AHE) is appropriate for enhancing local contrast. However, AHE has a propensity to enhance noise excessively. The over-amplification of noise that was caused by adaptive histogram equalization was the primary motivation for the development of CLAHE. This may be accomplished by controlling the amount of contrast enhancement that AHE provides.

3.2.2 Gaussian Filter

The CLAHE chest X-ray images are then passes through the Gaussian filter. Gaussian filters [15] are a type of linear smoothing filters that are effective at eliminating noise derived from a normal distribution. The Gaussian function in 2D dimension is as follows:

$$G(i, j) = \frac{1}{2\pi\sigma^2} e^{\frac{-i^2+j^2}{2\sigma^2}} \qquad (1)$$

Where σ represent standard deviation.

3.3 Vision Transformer

The transformer is a modern architecture in the field of natural language processing that intends to tackle sequence-to-sequence problems while also simplifying the process of dealing with long-range dependencies. It is a high-capacity network architecture that depends on self-attention. The attention-based transformer architecture, which is common within the domain of natural language processing, is adapted in a deep neural model known as a vision transformer to make it appropriate for pattern recognition. While the primary components of the original transformer design were an encoder and a decoder. Encoders are the only component in the architecture of the vision transformer. Given an input image, we divided an image into patches. After converting the input image into patches, we use a process known as linear projection to convert the patches into feature vectors. Linear projection occurs at the vision transformer input stage, and all patches go through a linear projection layer to produce the Z vector.

$$x \in R^{H \times W \times C} \qquad (2)$$

Where x denotes the input image, $H \times W \times C$ denotes the height, width and C represents the number of channels.

$$x_p^{(i)} \in R^{H \times W \times C} \qquad (3)$$

Where $x \in \{1 \ldots N\}$, N represent the number of patches. Position embedding is as simple as adding unique position to the linear projection of each patch so that the vision transformer knows the arrangement of the sequence during training. Vision transformer (VIT) also introduces a learnable class embedding or token. VIT also assigns a positional embedding to this class embedding. The final layer feature vector corresponding to this learnable class embedding is used by the MLP head for classification. The most important part of vision transformer is the encoder. The Transformer encoder [16] comprises of layer norm to reduce the training time as well as stabilize the training and Multi-Head self-attention (MHSA) to improve the overall network performance, skip connection is then used after attention in multi-layer perceptron (MLP) blocks. In the last stage, the features corresponding to the class embedding goes through a multi-layer perceptron (MLP) head for classification. Attention is mathematically defined as a function of three variables, Query, Key and Value. The dot product of Query and Key is scaled by a normalizing factor which is simply the dimension of the Z vector. The normalized dot product is then converted into probabilities by the softmax function.

$$Attention(Q, K, V) = Softmax\left(\frac{QK^T}{\sqrt{d_k}}\right)V \qquad (4)$$

Where Q represent the feature of interest, K denotes the feature that may be relevant to the feature of interest, V represents the original feature to be scaled by probabilities and d_k denotes the normalization factor.

4 Experiment Analysis

The chest X-ray images were pre-processed using CLAHE and Gaussian filter. 60% of the dataset is devoted to training, 20% to validation and 20% to testing. The inceptionV3, MobileNet, and Vision Transformer(google/vit-base-patch16–224-in21k) models were pre-trained on a large dataset [17] in this research using transfer learning approaches, and the models were then finetuned. By analyzing the model performance and adjusting the parameter values, we established the values of several hyperparameters and fixed the hyperparameter that improved performance. Optimizers like Stochastic Gradient Descent (SGD) and Adaptive Moment Estimation (ADAM) were used. The learning rate of 1e-4 with the ADAM optimizer showed a significant increase in performance over SGD. ReduceLROnPlateau was used in VIT to monitor model performance and cut the learning rate when there was no progress for N epochs.

5 Evaluation Metrics

The most often employed evaluation measures for covid-19 classification are Accuracy, precision, Recall, Specificity, F1-score and ROC curve. They are computed using the following equations:

$$Accuracy(A) = \frac{TP(True + ve) + TN(True - ve)}{TP(True + ve) + TN(True - ve) + FP(False + ve) \div FN(False - ve)} \qquad (5)$$

$$Precision(P) = \frac{TP}{TP + FP} \qquad (6)$$

$$Recall(R) = \frac{TP}{TP + FN} \qquad (7)$$

$$Specificity = \frac{TN}{TN + FP} \qquad (8)$$

$$F1 - score = 2 \times \frac{P \times R}{P + R} \qquad (9)$$

6 Evaluation Metrics

Binary classification is performed on two distinct classes (covid-19, normal) using chest radiography dataset. The finetuned VIT model performed better in the suggested task, with an accuracy of 98% and ROC curve of 98.52%. The pre-trained CNN, Inception V3, and MobileNet achieved 96% and 95% accuracy and ROC curve of 96.29% and 95.20% respectively. Figure 2 depicts the model confusion Matrix where 15 covid-19 images are misclassified as normal (false negative) and 7 normal chest X-ray images are misidentified as covid-19. ROC indicates the degree to which the model is able to differentiate between different classes. Figures 3, 4 and 5 represent the ROC Curve of the finetuned VIT model, Inception V3 and MobileNet. Table 1 represents the model specific efficiency metrics.

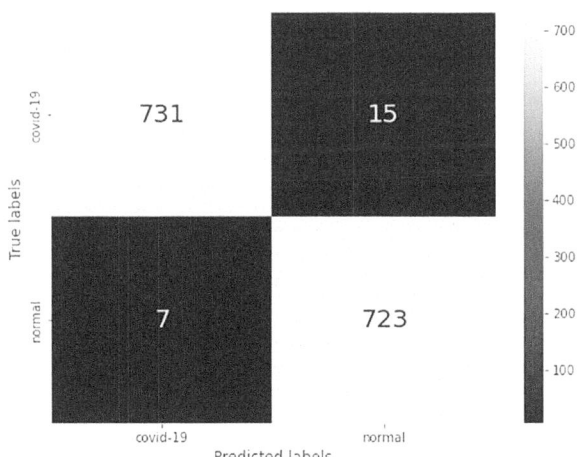

Fig. 2. Confusion matrix of finetuned Vision Transformer (VIT)

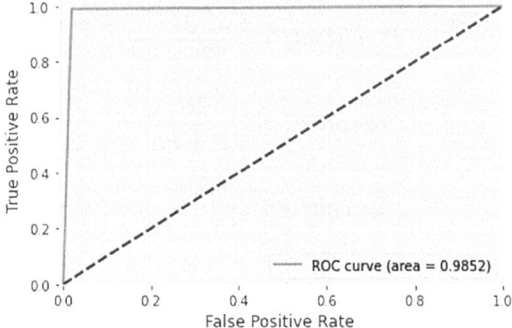

Fig. 3. ROC curve of finetuned Vision Transformer (VIT)

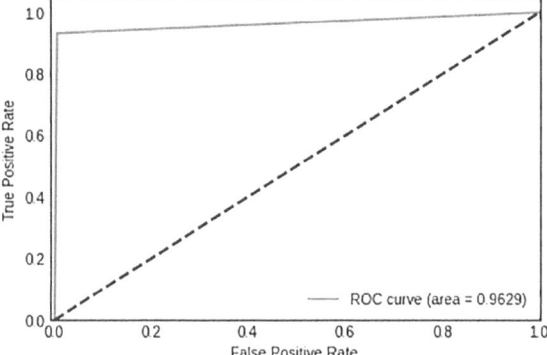

Fig. 4. ROC curve of Inception V3

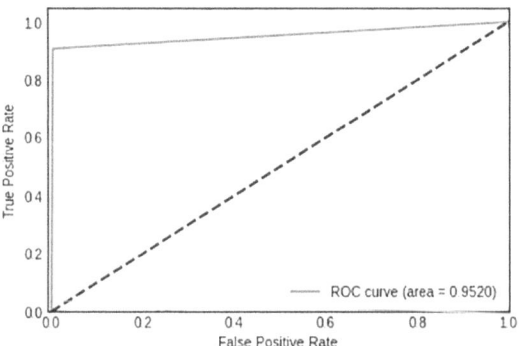

Fig. 5. ROC curve of MobileNet

Table 1. Model specific efficiency metrics

Model	Class	Precision(P)	Recall(R)	F1-score	Accuracy(A)
Inception V3	covid-19	0.94	0.99	0.96	0.96
	normal	0.99	0.93	0.96	
MobileNet	covid-19	0.92	1.00	0.95	0.95
	normal	1.00	0.91	0.95	
Finetuned VIT	covid-19	0.99	0.98	0.99	0.98
	normal	0.98	0.99	0.99	

7 Conclusion

The prompt and precise diagnosis of highly infectious covid-19 is an essential component in the overall strategy for controlling the virus further dissemination. Image enhancement techniques such as CLAHE and Gaussian filter were performed and the Vision Transformer is then finetuned. The finetuned VIT model performance is found to perform better when compared with SOTA convolutional neural network such as Inception V3 and MobileNet. In the future, this work might be expanded by presenting a segmentation-based technique for extracting more information from medical images.

References

1. de Santana, M.A., et al.: An intelligent tool to support diagnosis of Covid-19 by texture analysis of computerized tomography X-ray images and machine learning. In: Pani, S.K., Dash, S., dos Santos, W.P., Chan Bukhari, S.A., Flammini, F. (eds.) Assessing COVID-19 and Other Pandemics and Epidemics using Computational Modelling and Data Analysis, pp. 259–282. Springer, Cham (2022). https://doi.org/10.1007/978-3-030-79753-9_15
2. Abraham, B., Nair, M.S.: Computer-aided detection of COVID-19 from X-ray images using multi-CNN and Bayesnet classifier. Biocybernet. Biomed. Eng. **40**(4), 1436–1445 (2020)
3. Abbasian Ardakani, A., Acharya, U.R., Habibollahi, S., Mohammadi, A.: Covidiag: a clinical cad system to diagnose covid-19 pneumonia based on CT findings. Eur. Radiol. **31**(1), 121–130 (2021)
4. Rahman, M.M., Nooruddin, S., Hasan, K.M.A., Dey, N.K.: Hog + CNN net: diagnosing covid-19 and Pneumonia by deep neural network from chest x-ray images. SN Compu. Sci. **2**(5), 1–15 (2021)
5. Panwar, H., Gupta, P.K., Siddiqui, M.K., Morales-Menendez, R., Singh, V.: Application of deep learning for fast detection of covid-19 in X-Rays using ncovnet. Chaos Solitons Fractals **138**, 109944 (2020)
6. Mondal, A.K., Bhattacharjee, A., Singla, P., Prathosh, A.P.: XViTCOS: Explainable vision transformer based COVID-19 screening using radiography. IEEE J. Trans. Eng. Health Med. **10**, 1–10 (2022)
7. Dilshad, S., et al.: Automated image classification of chest x-rays of covid-19 using deep transfer learning. Results Phys. **28**, 104529 (2021). https://doi.org/10.1016/J.RINP.2021.104529

8. Narin, A., Kaya, C., Pamuk, Z.: Automatic detection of coronavirus disease (COVID-19) using X-ray images and deep convolutional neural networks. Patt. Anal. Appl. **24**(3), 1207–1220 (2020)
9. Minaee, S., Kafieh, R., Sonka, M., Yazdani, S., Jamalipour Soufi, G.: Deep-COVID: predicting COVID-19 from chest X-ray images using deep transfer learning. Med. Image Anal. **65**, 101794 (2020)
10. Wang, C., et al.: Pulmonary image classification based on inception-v3 transfer learning model. IEEE Access **7**, 146533–146541 (2019)
11. Howard, A.G., et al.: MobileNets: Efficient Convolutional Neural Networks for Mobile Vision Applications (2017)
12. Dosovitskiy, A., et al.: An image is worth 16x16 words: Transformers for image recognition at scale. arXiv preprint arXiv:2010.11929 (2020)
13. Chowdhury, M.E.H., et al.: Can AI help in screening viral and COVID-19 pneumonia? IEEE Access **8**, 132665–132676 (2020). https://doi.org/10.1109/ACCESS.2020.3010287
14. Rahman, T., et al.: Exploring the effect of image enhancement techniques on COVID-19 detection using chest X-ray images. Comput. Biol. Med. **132**, 104319 (2021)
15. Punitha, S., Amuthan, A., Joseph, K.S.: Benign and malignant breast cancer segmentation using optimized region growing technique. Future Comput. Inform. J. **3**(2), 348–358 (2018)
16. Vaswani, A., et al.: Attention is all you need. Adv. Neural Inform. Process. Syst. **30** (2017)
17. Deng, J., Dong, W., Socher, R., Li, L.-J., Li, K., Fei-Fei, L.: ImageNet: a large-scale hierarchical image database. In: IEEE Conference on Computer Vision and Pattern Recognition, pp. 248–255 (2010)

Performance Analysis of Classification and Boosting Algorithm for Diabetes Prediction

Shekharesh Barik[✉], Chandan Kumar Behera, Pravat Kumar Behera, and Subhranshu Nanda Brahmachary

Department of CSE, DRIEMS (Autonomous), Cuttack, Odisha, India
shekharesh@gmail.com

Abstract. In the world more than 400 million people are suffering in diabetes. One of the most vital health disabilities is diabetes in Modern times . Diabetes is a condition in which the body's glucose levels rise above normal. It is a chronic disorder that interferes the system of the body regulates the blood sugar. Diabetes can lead to various complications like visual impairment, kidney disappointment, cardiovascular breakdown and stroke. Now a days, people of different age groups are affected with diabetes. Diabetes can attack to younger as well as older persons. Early diagnosis of diabetes is extremely urgent so as to spare individual from diabetes . All known that diabetes is of two types, these are Type1 and Type2; even there are also sensory sorts, for an example mutation diabetes, which occurs during pregnant. Machine Learning algorithm can assist in detecting the diabetes mellitus. This method aids in boosting diagnostic accuracy while lowering the price of medical supplies. Patient health risk can be decreased by early diabetes identification. The result of the prediction can be useful information to the specialists, patients and patients 'family members. Due to limited healthcare resources, it is required to anticipate the patient's current health status after admission. Large volumes of data have been produced by mean of extensive analysis into every area of diabetes (diagnosis, therapy, etc.). Finding the right pattern in a large dataset is an issue of information processing. This encourages us to construct certain end out of accessible dataset. The scientific procedure should be possible by various Machine learning procedures. This paper gives an insight into the ongoing improvements in ML for recognition and determination of diabetes. Recent advancements in ML have been fruitful at anticipating diabetes from the therapeutic past of the diabetic patient. Notwithstanding, these methodologies depend on an enormous number of clinical factors in this way requiring machine learning procedures. Five numbers of algorithms are explained here. These algorithms were actualized and contrasted all together with investigate the forecast exactness for diabetes. At long last, we think about every one of these comparison results and pick the effective one according to its precision level.

Keywords: Medical diagnosis · Clinical factors · Comparative analysis

1 Introduction

The metabolic disorders collectively referred to as "diabetes" are known to have a significant negative impact on human health globally. Patients with diabetes have a wide range of high-risk factors, and many of them experience complications and harm that could be prevented. To lower the frequency of problems, the level of high-risk factor detection might be raised. As a result, we must examine a person's complete medical and health history, which currently requires medical professionals and is labor-intensive, subjective, and manual. In this study, our aim is to assess a collection of algorithms that perform well for predicting diabetes. In the modern world, diabetes is one of India's biggest health problems. It is a collection of ailments brought on by excessive blood sugar levels. Increased appetite, extreme/frequent urination, extreme thirst, tiredness, vision problems, loss of weight, mood fluctuations, confusion, and concentration difficulties are just a few of the symptoms of diabetes. It can also lead to recurrent infections and a slow recovery. Basically, Type 1 diabetes, attacks the pancreatic beta cells (autoimmunity) or the body's immune system damages. A high blood sugar level forms from this attack because the beta cells cannot produce the necessary quantity of insulin to transport glucose into the cells because they die (hyperglycemia). Type 1 diabetes, which often affects those under 30 but can strike anybody at any age, accounts for 5–10% of all cases of diabetes. The symptoms generally appear quickly and are severe. Because Type I diabetes is characterized by a shortage of insulin, patients must supplement what the body cannot manufacture. People generally neglect type 1 diabetes until serious symptoms emerge and hospitalization is necessary. Diabetes can lead to a multitude of health issues if neglected. That is why it is critical to be aware of the warning signals and to contact a healthcare professional on a regular basis for routine wellness checks.

Computers are intelligent machines that can be trained to make decisions in the same way that humans do. There are many kinds of systems gaining knowledge of techniques that are used to categorize the statistics units. These are supervised, deep learning, evolutionary learning, Unsupervised Reinforcement, and semi-surveyed Diabetes prevention and prediction are topics that the medical sciences are growing more and more interested in. The objective is to use a variety of machine learning techniques to predict diabetes early on. In this research, we mostly use well-known classifiers like the decision tree. K-Nearest Neighbors, support vector machine and Random Forest. Most of these category strategies are implemented on the Pima Indian diabetes dataset. As a result, we can predict diabetes with the aid of considering numerous sets of degrees and examining the performance of diverse category strategies. Additionally, utilizing boosting machine learning methods like Adaboost, we provided a conceptual model for the prediction of diabetes type 5 Mellitus. We examine the accuracy of fifty-four exceptional devices, getting to know technology, to locate diabetes at an early stage. The go-validation approach is used for feature choice. The capabilities thus received are used with exclusive ML classifiers [1, 3].

Machine learning strategies, such as KNN, Random forest and decision trees were employed. A random forest model was claimed to have an accuracy of 75.11%, a decision tree model 71.08%, and the K Nearest Neighbour (KNN) method of 76.7%. Adaboost with the help of Vector Machines (SVM) as base estimators have also been used. Those methods have implemented the use of Python programming tools. The maximum accuracy obtained among those classifiers is 76.7%.

2 Related Work

Diabetes may be a condition that happens once the blood glucose level is simply too high. A diabetic should routinely check their blood sugar level. When his sugar level reaches or exceeds the normal range, he should take precautions. Diabetes patients are at risk for major health issues in the future. Diabetes causes the patient to develop cardiovascular and other problems. Additionally, it has been noted that these issues disrupt the family's overall financial, psychological, and economic equilibrium According to a research by the International Diabetes Federation, there will be 380 million diabetics globally in the next 20 years. Given its importance, diabetes must be recognized more accurately and at lower cost. Different machine learning algorithms have been tested by researchers in an effort to produce reliable findings for illness prevention [2].

Negi et al. have used the Support Vector Machine (SVM) algorithm to analyze and predict diabetes. Two datasets that are used are PIMA Indians dataset and 130-US dataset. The objective of combining the datasets is to get a reliable dataset. After combining, the number of samples became 102,538 samples and number of attributes became 49. Out of these, 64,419 samples were positive, and 38,115 Samples were negative. Different feature selection techniques were employed before the model was implemented. LIB-SVM package is used which selects four attributes. In addition, WEKA tool is also used which selects 20 attributes. Cross validation technique is used for efficient validation of the dataset. The combination of two datasets offers a reliable result, with an accuracy of 72% [4].

Several supervised machine learning techniques, as well as Levenberg-Marquardt (LM), Bayesian Regulation (BR) and Scaled Conjugate Gradient (SCG) were used by Mamuda et al. (SCG) [5]. The Pima Indian dataset was used to test the performance (768 samples and eight attributes). To validate the dataset, they used the cross validation method, which divides it into training and testing sets. Levenberg Marquardt (LM), according to the authors, had the best validation set performance, with a Mean Squared Error (MSE) of 0.00025091.

In his study, Yun Sheng used DISKR and the KNN approach to eliminate outliers and OOBs (out of bag) (Reduce the size of the K-nearest neighbours training set.). The space complexity diminishes, the researchers' accuracy increases, and the researchers' results are improved after removing factors or instances that have little bearing [6].

Diabetes was identified by Deepti et al. using Naive Bayes classifiers, decision tree and support vector machine (SVM). They have utilized the Pima Indian Dataset to apply the model B in order to find the maximum reliability or accuracy. Cross-validation is a method that is used to segment the dataset into sets. The author doesn't address data preparation. Accuracy, the F measure, recall, and other performance metrics are used to assess the algorithm's effectiveness. The Naive Bayes model has the highest accuracy (76.30%) [7].

The goal of B. Tamilvanan et al. to figure diabetes more precisely. The exactness rates of the three classification calculations —decision tree, Random Forest and Naive

Bayes—are compared. The WEKA tool is used for implementation. As a result, Naive Bayes has the lowest error rate (23.7%) and the highest predictive capability (76.3%) [8].

Using the Pima Indian Diabetes datasets, Monisha. A et al. assess a number of classifiers, including logistical regression, Extreme Gradient Boosting and Naive Bayes statistical modeling in order to predict and diagnose diabetes. With an 81% accuracy rate, the Extreme Gradient Boosting method performs better than the other two methods [9].

Yuvraj et al. demonstrated a model of diabetes prediction by using three distinct Machine Learning algorithms such as Decision tree, Naïve Bayes and Random Forest after eliminating the null values by pre-processing. The detail of pre-processed was not discussed by the authors. In order to extract relevant features, form the dataset, Information Gain method is used. Among 13 attributes, 8 attributes are selected by feature selection method. To continue the proper study, they have divided the dataset into two sets such as 70% of the data are reserved as the training data set and 30% of the data are reserved as the test dataset. They have succeeded in discovering the accuracy rate of 94% in which the Random Forest algorithm performs well enough [10].

Challenges related to diabetes were explored by S. Selvakumar et al. To determine if a person has diabetes or not, multilayer perception, the K-Nearest Neighbor method binary logistic regression are employed. Multilayer Perception's accuracy level is 0.71, Binary Logistic Regression's accuracy level is 0.69, and K-Nearest Neighbor's accuracy level is 0.80. The most accurate of these is K Nearest Neighbour, followed by Multilayer Perception and Binary Logistic Regression [11].

Soltani et al. shows in a study that they used the (PNN) Probabilistic Neural Network to detect diabetes. The dataset for PIMA Indians was appeal to the algorithm. Any pre-processing technique didn't apply by the authors. The entire dataset is spitted in training and testing set with a ration 9:1. For the training and testing sets of data, the suggested method's accuracy was 89.56% and 81.49%, respectively [12].

Deepika Verma et al. take two disease datasets. These are diabetic and breast cancer datasets from the machine learning repository at UCI. This research uses the effective classification that is WEKA Algorithm tool. Using the WEKA interface, SMO, REP tree, j48, Naive Bayes and MLP algorithms were used to classify a dataset for diabetes and breast cancer. After prediction the performance of all algorithms, from diabetes datasets SMO achieves 76.80% accuracy level and J48 gets 74.28% accuracy level than the other algorithms on breast cancer dataset [13].

Kandhasamy et al. applied a number of classifiers SVM, j48, (KNN) K-Nearest Neighbors and Random Forest. The dataset is collected from UCI repository over which the ML algorithms were performed. A comparison of algorithms was carried out with respect to result accuracy, specificity and sensitivity. The classification is done after pre-processing of data and also without pre-processing on the data. For validation, cross validation technique is used. Pre-processing is done by removing noise from the data. Without pre-processing, Decision tree come up with highest accuracy rate that is 73.82%. But, KNN (k = 1) algorithm and after pre-processing Random Forest algorithm provided highest accuracy rate of 100% [14].

Rahul Joshi et al. say that prediction using machine learning techniques from early dataset development is safe for human life. To predict diabetes WEKA and java tools. Random Forest, Naive Bayes, KNNand J48 are the applied algorithms. The best result is found in collected approach, which combines individual methods and techniques. It is also named as hybrid model. This gives the improved accuracy and performance compared to using a single one [15].

Mercaldo et al. six different types of classifiers are used. These are J48, Hoeffding Tree, Multilayer Perceptron, Bayes, JRip and Random Forest. For this study, the Pima Indian dataset was also used.. In order to increase the performance of classification, two algorithms, Greedy and Best First, were used which 40 in determine the discriminatory attributes. The attributes which were selected are diabetes pedigree function, body mass index, plasma glucose concentration and age. They have used cross validation for 48 lation of the dataset. All the classifier algorithms were compared by taking the parameters like F-Measure, recall, precision. The Hoeffding Tree algorithm provided precision value as 0.757, F-measure value as 0.759 and recall value as to 0.762. This was the highest performance in comparison to the other algorithms [16].

S M Hasan Mahmud et al. determine the diabetes' state. The five most vital machine learning classification algorithms for predicting diabetes were examined in this article. Methods of 10-fold cross validation were used to see how well the categorization approaches performed. The analysis's findings demonstrate that Naive Bayes, which obtained an F1 score of 0.74, outperformed the other classifiers in terms of performance [17].

Tafa et al. projected a replacement integrated improved model of SVM and Naïve Thomas Bayes for predicting the polygenic disorder. Analysis of the model was done by a dataset that was collected from completely different regions in Kosovo. There have been eight attributes within the data's and 402 rows. From these, eighty numbers of rows or patients were full of sort two polygenic disorder. Some attributes used during this study haven't been investigated before, as well as the regular twenty three physical activity, and case history of polygenic disorder. To perform validation, the dataset was divided into coaching set associated testing set with an magnitude relation of 50:50. The algorithms gave a really sensible performance with a prediction accuracy of ninety seven.6%, wherever because the performance of SVM and Naïve Thomas Bayes was ninety five.52% and 94.52%, severally [18].

Xue-huimeng et al. compare three algorithms to predict diabetes by using similar risk indicators. 735 patients from two villages in Guangzhou, China, were tested using the logistic30 algorithm, ANN, and decision tree algorithms. The classification algorithm achieves the maximum degree of accuracy (77.87%). (C5.0) [19].

Amina Azar et al. say both young individuals and ancient peoples were impacted by diabetes. These are getting worse every day and there is no cure. Early stage prediction is achieved by data mining. The primary goals of this work are to provide distinction and recommend the optimal algorithm. We employ the PID datasets. With the maximum accuracy and effectiveness, (KNN) K-Nearest Neighbor, Naïve Bayes and the Decision Tree algorithms are evaluated and utilized to predict the early diagnosis of diabetes. Rapid Miner is used to test and validate the WEKA. The decision tree is shown to be the most reliable prediction technique. The accuracy level is 75.65% [20].

Aiswarya Iyaret al. Uses decision trees and simple Bayesian algorithms to find solutions for diagnosing diseases. For implementation the WEKA tool is used. 79.56% accuracy achieved the Naive Bayes algorithm [21].

Deepti Sisodia et al. work 43 diabetes prediction at early stage. Accuracy is evaluated using WEKA tool. For prediction Naïve Bayes, support vector machine (SVM) and Decision tree classification algorithms are used. The Naïve Bayes gave the highest accuracy [22].

Aakansha Rathore et al. find and anticipate diabetes disease. Diabetes dataset for Pima Indians was used experimentally, and R Studio was used to assess the performance measures. SVM and Decision Tree are two machine learning techniques that are employed. The accuracy of the SV is 82% [23].

Olaniyi et al. implement a multilayer feed-forward neural network. Back-propagation technique was used to complete 36 training. The PIMA Indian Diabetes database was utilized to apply the algorithms. Prior to processing, the dataset is normalized to ensure numerical stability. It involves swapping out amplitude ranges of 0 to 1. 500 samples from the whole dataset were utilized for the training set, while 268 samples were used for the testing set. The accuracy rate of 82% that was attained is seen to be high [24].

3 Analysis of Dataset

The patient dataset is used to predict the class to which a patient belongs. The classification is binary (0 or 1). That means the outcome of prediction will say whether a patient has developed diabetics or not. The dataset used for this categorization purpose National Institute of Diabetes and Digestive and Kidney Diseases which is provide PIMA Diabetes dataset. The data set contains 768 number of rows and 9 number of columns. Hence, we have with us 9 features or attributes. These features are named as: Pregnancies, Age, Glucose, BMI, Blood Pressure, Insulin, SkinThickness, DiabetesPedigreeFunction, and outcomes.

To build a model that can predict or identify whether a man is a diabetes patient or not. We have implemented five machine learning algorithms like (KNN)K-Nearest Neighbor, Adaboost with Support Vector Machine (SVM),Decision Tree (DT), and Adaboost with the Decision Tree algorithm. The machine learning methods outlined above were implemented using the Python programming language. The data is saved as a CSV file. We imported the Pandas module as a data frame to integrate the data into our software. Then we may execute numerous data analysis processes. We also need to load modules like Numpy to analyze the data. Now a day's using machine learning methods diabetes has predicted. To plot any form of graph, we must first import the Matplotlib package. We may see the data in graphical representation by using this module. We utilized cross-validation to locate the proper pattern in the dataset.

4 Methodology

4.1 Decision Tree

Various factors are used to form a decision tree. It falls under the category of guided learning. By learning certain decision-making principles, we forecast the objective. These also rely on the characteristics of the data. Similar to if-then-else statements, decision rules are statements. A tree's node functions as a test case for an attribute. One of the solutions for the test case is represented by the tree edge. Apply the decision rules to a specific instance of the problem to use the decision tree to classify the issue from root to leaf node. The label or output is represented by the leaf nodes [25]. We must import the Decision Tree Classifier from the two Sklearn modules in order to create the decision tree method. The next stage is to split the data set into training and testing. To improve the predictive accuracy of the algorithm, cross validation was used. A random seed is necessary for the operation of a decision tree. This setting regulates the random selections. This is an arbitrary number. The random state in this situation is 7. The cross fold value we used was cv 10. This shows that there are 10 components to the overall dataset. It requires nine of them for training and one for testing. In order to cover the whole data set, this process is performed on a random basis. Prediction value is calculated by finding the mean of all scores. Here, we found the prediction value 0.710885.

4.2 Random Forest Classifier

The supervised learning method known as Random Forest is frequently used to solve classification problems. As far as we all know, a forest is made up of trees. Similar to that, it creates a variety of decision trees using the data samples. Each decision tree randomly selects a dataset feature to represent. Each tree provides a value for prediction. The voting procedure is used to determine the final decision value or the best value. The vote is the process which finds the most voted prediction value. Decision tree reduces the over fitting problem. Here we have calculated the output by finding the mean of all prediction scores. Random forest overcomes high variance and low bias problem which is found in case of decision trees. But random forest may be slower in comparison to decision tree. It has a greater number of decision trees [26]. Our dataset, we must import the Random Forest classifier in order to build it. The sklearn module's Random Forest 25 class is a classifier. We've broken up. Training and testing groups using the dataset. Approximately 70% of the whole dataset is used for training and 30 percent are tests. Now that the n-estimator is present, we can use the Random Forest classifier.value is 10, and the n-estimator denotes how many decision trees will be built throughout the operation. Random forest comes with the accuracy of 75.11%. This accuracy value can be improved by adjusting different hyper parameters.

4.3 K-Nearest Neighbor (K-NN)

K-Nearest Neighbor (KNN) is a supervised learning algorithm that's mainly used for type issues. It is simple to implement this version from a dataset. KNN does no longer have a special schooling section. So it's miles taken into consideration as a lazy learning algorithm. Here k represents the quantity nearest friends. KNN algorithms classify new information points based totally on similarity measures (e.g. distance characteristic). Class is in line with most people of balloting to buddies. Data is sent to the class with the closest neighbors. If k's numerical value is raised. Prediction accuracy might improve. Finding the ideal k value for the given data collection is a challenging issue. From one dataset to the next, the k value will change. This model's governing variable is the value of k. The suitable value of k must be used. An issue with over fitting may develop if we choose a smaller value of k [27] the calculations become more complex if we choose a higher value for k. By running the opera on several values of k, we have improved the process of determining the value of k. The best k value is then selected based on the results. A distance metric is used to identify which of the k instances in the training dataset are comparable to a new input. The generally used approach is Euclidean distance. 35 If x is a new point (x) and xi is an existing point across all input characteristics (j), then the distance between these two can be expressed as follows:

$$d(x, xi) = \sqrt{(xi - xij)^2} \tag{1}$$

To implement the KNN classifier in our program, we have to import Sklearn module then we have to convert the categorical variables to numeric variables. We have studied the performance over a range of K values to find the best and suitable values of K. For our model, we have taken k value in a range of (1, 21). Cross validation method is used for accurate measure of the performance of this model [28].

We found the k value is highest at k = 18, so this value of k is chosen and then applied to the KNN classifier. We get the prediction accuracy of 76.7%.

5 Results and Comparison

We are using particular sorts of matrices like confusion matrix, accuracy, and F1 score to compare the results of the various models we have developed. Confusion score provides a more realistic picture of the model's performance. The Confusion matrix, a two-dimensional array, includes the phrases True Negative, True Positive, False Negative and False Positive [29] (Fig. 1).

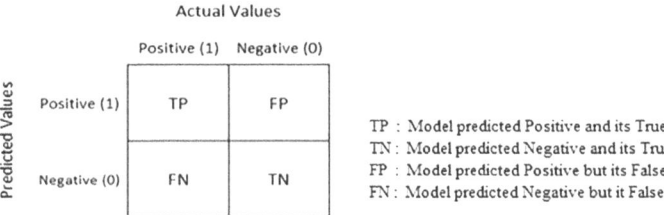

Fig. 1. Four outcomes of Confusion Matrix

$$F - measure = \frac{2 * recall * precision}{recall + precision}$$

The F1 Score is a statistic that provides us with precise model information. It strikes a balance between accuracy and memory. F1 score is significant because it may be used to simultaneously quantify recall and accuracy using a harmonic mean.

On our dataset, we have applied five machine learning methods. Based on the prediction accuracy, all machine learning methods are taken into account in a comparative study. We discovered that the decision tree's prediction accuracy is 71.08%, the Random Forest's is 75.11%, and the K-Nearest Neighbor (K-NN) method's is 76.7%. Adaboost with Support Vector Machines (SVM) yields 62.33%, whereas Adaboost with decision trees yields 74.45%. Therefore, it is evident that K-NN, with a resultant accuracy of 76.7%, is the classifier that achieves the highest accuracy (Table 1).

Table 1. Accuracy, and F1 Score for ML Algorithms

Algorithm Name	Accuracy	F1 score	Confusion Matrix
Decision Tree	0.7108	0.5889	[[116 28] [39 48]]
Random Forest	0.7511	0.5531	[[129 15] [48 39]]
KNN	0.7670	0.4822	[[124 20] [53 34]]
Adaboost with SVM	0.6233	0.5972	[[130 14] [44 43]]
Adaboost with DT	0.7455	0.6143	[[125 19] [40 47]]

By placing False Positive rate on the X-axis, True Positive rate on the Y-axis the AUC-ROC curve is created. AUC is a measurement of separability. The model performs better at differentiating between individuals with and without illness the higher the AUC (Figs. 2 and 3).

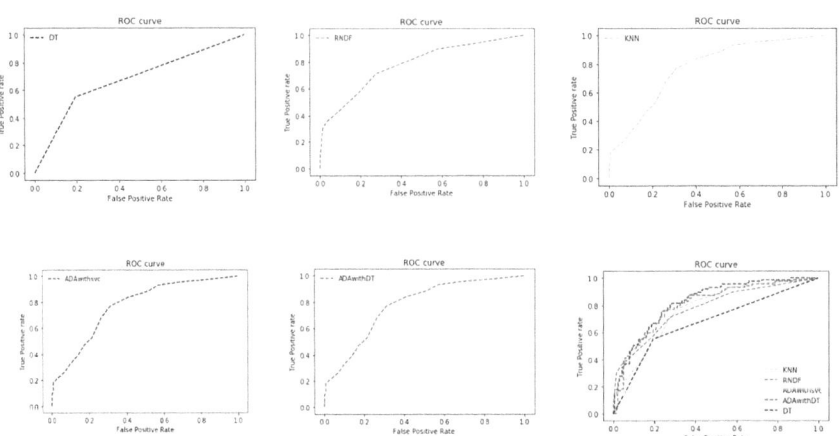

Fig. 2. AUC-ROC curve of Machine Learning algorithms and their comparisons

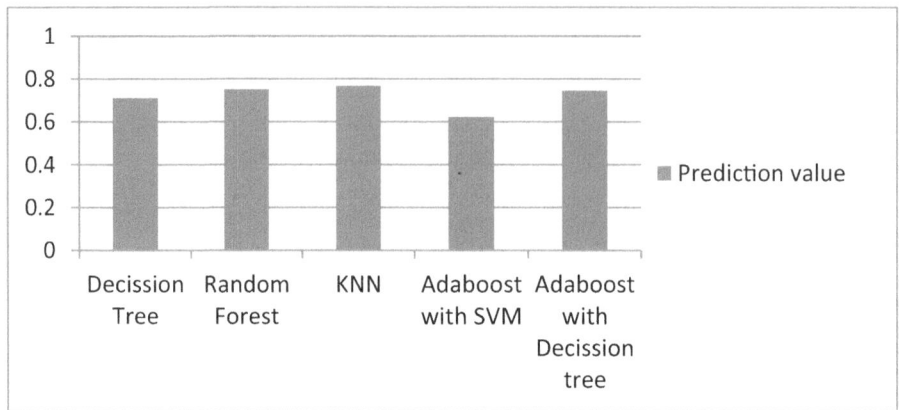

Fig. 3. Prediction Accuracy Results of Machine Learning Algorithms

6 Conclusion and Future Scope

Physicians and medical staff will find a useful answer from predictive analysis in the healthcare industry. They will undoubtedly benefit from this field's unique approach and better serve society by utilizing these machine learning techniques. using the dataset used in this study, we used five machine learning algorithms to estimate the accuracy value for diabetes. One of them, K Nearest Neighbor (K-NN), has a low-error diabetes prediction accuracy of 76.7%. By adjusting the hyper parameters or using an ensemble of additional classifiers, machine learning algorithms can further increase their accuracy. Additionally, the deployment of the aforementioned machine learning algorithms with new data might expand the scope of the aforementioned study activity.

References

1. Kaschel, H., Rocco, V., Reinao, G.: An open algorithm for systematic evaluation of readmission predictors on diabetic patients from data warehouses. In: 2018 IEEE International Conference on Automation/XXIIICongress of the Chilean Association of Automatic Control, pp. 1–6. IEEE (2018)
2. Chen, M., Hao, Y.K., Hwang, K., et al.: Disease prediction by machine learning over big data from healthcare communities. IEEE Access **5**, 8869–8879 (2017)
3. Baboota, R., Kaur, H.: Predictive analysis and modelling football results using machine learning approach for English Premier League. Int. J. Forecast. **35**(2), 741–755 (2019)
4. Negi, A., Jaiswal, V.: A first attempt to develop a diabetes prediction method based on different global datasets. In: Proceedings of the 2016 Fourth International Conference on Parallel, Distributed and Grid Computing (PDGC), Waknaghat, India, pp. 237–241, 22–24 December 2016
5. Mamuda, M., Sathasivam, S.: Predicting the survival of diabetes using neural network. In: Proceedings of the AIP Conference Proceedings, Bydgoszcz, Poland, vol. 1870, pp. 40–46, 9–11 May 2017
6. Sheng, Y., Liang, J., Lu, J., Zhao, X.: An efficient instance selection algorithm for k nearest neighbour regression. Neuro Comput. **251**, 26–34 (2017)

7. Sisodia, D., Sisodia, D.S.: Prediction of diabetes using classification algorithm. Proc. Comput. Sci. **132**, 1578–1585 (2018). www.elsevier.com/locate/procedia
8. Tamilvanan, B., MuraliBhaskaran, V.: An experimental study of diabetes disease prediction system using classification techniques. IOSR J. Comput. Eng. (IOSR-JCE) **19**(1), Ver. IV, 39–44, January–February 2017. e-ISSN: 2278-0661, ISSN: 2278-8727
9. Monisha, A., Shalin Chistina, S., Santiago, N.: Decision support system for a chronic disease-Diabetes. Int. J. Comput. Mathe. Sci. (IJCMS), **7**(3), March 2018. ISSN 2347-8527
10. Yuvaraj, N., Sri Preethaa, K.R.: Diabetes prediction in healthcare systems using machine learning algorithms on Hadoop cluster. Clust. Comput. **22**, 1–9 (2017)
11. Selvakumar, S., Senthamarai Kannan, K., Gothai Nachiyar, S.: Prediction of diabetes diagnosis using classification based data mining techniques. Int. J. Stat. Syst. **12**(2), 183–188 (2017). ISSN 0973-2675
12. Soltani, Z., Jafarian, A.: A new artificial neural networks approach for diagnosing diabetes disease type II. Int. J. Adv. Comput. Sci. Appl. **7**, 89–94 (2016)
13. Verma, D., Mishra, N.: Analysis and prediction of breast cancer and diabetes disease dataset using data mining classification techniques. In: Proceedings of the International Conference on Intelligent Sustainable Systems (ICISS 2017), IEEE Xplore Compliant - Part Number:CFP17M19-ART. ISBN:978-1-5386-1959-9
14. Kandhasamy, J.P., Balamurali, S.: Performance analysis of classifier models to predict diabetes mellitus. Proc. Comput. Sci. **47**, 45–51 (2015)
15. Joshi, R., Alehegn, M.: Analysis and prediction of diabetes diseases using machine learning algorithm: Ensemble approach. Int. Res. J. Eng. Technol. (IRJET), **04**(10), October 2017. e-ISSN: 2395-0056, p-ISSN: 2395-0072
16. Mercaldo, F., Nardone, V., Santone, A.: Diabetes mellitus affected patients classification and diagnosis through machine learning techniques. Proc. Comput. Sci. **112**, 2519–2528 (2017)
17. Hasan Mahmud, S.M., Hossin, M.A., Ahmed, M.R., Haider Noori, S.R., Islam Sarkar, M.N.: Machine learning based unified framework for diabetes prediction. In: BDET 2018, 25–27 August 2018, Chengdu, China (2018). © 2018 Association for Computing Machinery. ACM ISBN 978-1-4503-6582, 6/18/08. https://doi.org/10.1145/3297730.3297737
18. Tafa, Z., Pervetica, N., Karahoda, B.: An intelligent system for diabetes prediction. In: Proceedings of the 2015 4th Mediterranean Conference on Embedded Computing (MECO), Budva, Montenegro, 14–18 June 2015, pp. 378–382 (2015)
19. Menget, X.-H., Huang, Y.-X., Rao, D.-P., Liu, Q.: Comparison of three data mining models for predicting diabetes of prediabetes by risk factors. Kaohsiung J. Med. Sci. **29**, 93–99 (2013)
20. Azar, A., Ali, Y., Awais, M., Zaheer, K.: Data mining models comparison for diabetes prediction. (IJACSA) Int. J. Adv. Comput. Sci. Appl. **9**(8) (2018)
21. Iyar, A., Jeyalatha, S., Sumbaly, R.: Diagnosis of diabetes using classification mining techniques. Int. J. Data Min. Knowl. Manag. Process (IJDKP) **5**(1), January 2015
22. Sisodia, D., Sisodia, D.S.: Prediction of diabetes using classification algorithms. Proc. Comput. Sci. **132**, 1578–1585 (2018)
23. Rathore, A., Chauhan, S., Gujral, S.: Detecting and predicting diabetes using supervised learning: an approach towards better healthcare for Women. **8**(5), May–June 2017. ISSN No. 0976-5697
24. Olaniyi, E.O., Adnan, K.: Onset diabetes diagnosis using artificial neural network. Int. J. Sci. Eng. Res. **5**, 754–759 (2014)
25. Vijayan, V., Ravi, K.: Prediction and diagnosis of diabetes mellitus—a machine learning approach, pp 122–127, December 2015
26. Georga, E., et al.: Data mining for blood glucose prediction and knowledge discovery in diabetic patients: the METABO diabetes modeling and management system. In: 31st Annual International Conference, IEEE EMBS Minneapolis, Minnesota, USA, vol. 43100, pp. 5633–5636 (2009)

27. Zhang, D., Wang, X.: An optimized tongue image color correction scheme. IEEE Trans. Inf. Technol. Biomed. **14**(6), 1355–1364 (2010)
28. Kavakiotis, I., Tsave, O., Salifoglou, A., Maglaveras, N., Vlahavas, I., Chouvarda, I.: Machine learning and data mining methods in diabetes research. Comput. Struct. Biotechnol. J. **15**, 104–116 (2017). https://doi.org/10.1016/j.csbj.2016.12.005
29. Park, S., Choi, D., Kim, M., Cha, W., Kim, C., Moon, I.C.: Identifying prescription patterns with a topic model of diseases and medications. J. Biomed. Informat. **75**, 35–47 (2017)

An ISDUMD Algorithm Using Bayesian Averaging for Smoothing 3D Reconstruction of 2D MRI Medical Images

Mriganka Sarmah[1(✉)], Arambam Neelima[1], and Puspakshi Sarmah[2]

[1] CSE, NIT, Dimapur, Nagaland 797103, India
mrigankasarmahcse@gmail.com
[2] CS, NEF College, Guwahati, Assam 781040, India

Abstract. 3D reconstruction from 2D medical images is a challenging approximation method due to the unavailability of point normal. Medical 3D models are generated using Marching Cube (MC) algorithm but it generates a rough and ugly surface mesh. Mesh denoising is done to smooth the noise using many techniques such as Laplacian, Humphrey's Class (HC), Mean Curvature Flow (MCF), Taubin's signal processing approach, and Scale Dependant Umbrella (SDU). In this paper, an improved scale dependant umbrella mesh denoising algorithm (ISDUMD) is proposed that corrects the SDU algorithm up to 4.21% using the Bayesian Averaging Method (BAM). BAM is used to determine the average of a distribution from a predetermined average. The constant 'c' in the BAM is experimentally determined at 0.001. The proposed ISDUMD (SDU + BAM) method had 4.03\% less volume shrinkage as compared to SDU and 7.12% better Structural Similarity Index Measure (SSIM) score than SDU after 10 iterations. The test is done on a brain model with synthetically added 33.217 dB PSNR random noise. The dataset used is UPENN-GBM and is openly available.

Keywords: 3D reconstruction · mesh denoising · surface smoothing · Bayesian averaging · marching cube

1 Introduction

Mesh smoothing [1] is a technique to remove noisy vertex locations to a new position such that a smooth texture is rendered to the 3D model. These mesh vertices are acquired from key-point locations [2] on 2D medical scans. The region of interest of the organ thereafter needs to be segmented and registered to a common reference frame [3]. The segmentation [4] is a semi-automatic process and thus the produced regions have rough edges which needs some post-processing before rendering the final 3D shape. Human internal organs are only visible through radiographic imaging, and for a single patient variable number of slices are generated as a 2D image. These slices are understood by medical professionals only, but in modern times, the need for a 3D model of the internal organs is rising both for the medical professionals and patient as these 3D reconstruction gives a better representation of the surrounding areas of the affected organ. As the 3D models are developed, the accuracy of the organ is also important. Radiologists use high-resolution computed tomography (HRCT), magnetic resonance imaging (MRI), and functional magnetic resonance imaging (fMRI) to diagnose complex diseases. While using these modalities the organs, tissues, fat, and other fluids in the vicinity of the organ of interest produce unwanted information causing irregular surface texture [5]. These small stains and noise are not visible in the scans until the 3D model is reconstructed. On the other hand, segmentation error [6] can cause missing information and render a noisy depression over the organ tissue which is not a part of the ground truth. The 3D models are represented as a polygonal mesh. Each polygon is described by the vertices and the edges connecting the vertices. Sometimes additional information is also provided such as vertex normal, vertex texture and colour. Mesh smoothing is the iterative process of converging a noisy vertex to an optimum vertex location such that the neighbourhood tends to be as smooth as possible. The noisy vertex tends to be pulling the surface outwards or inwards causing a surface artifact. The initial structure of the mesh is generated using the marching cube algorithm [7] but, the overall model quality is not good. And hence the surface smoothing is needed. Some widely used mesh denoising algorithms are Laplacian [8], improved Laplacian [9], Taubin's signal processing approach [10], mean curvature flow (MCF) [11], and scale dependant umbrella (SDU) [12]. All of these methods are an iterative processes and converges based on the rate of smoothing, attributed to the smoothing factor. The SDU algorithm is a technique where the vertex locations are moved based on the edge length of the neighbouring vertex with the central vertex. Basically the inverse relation 1/edge causes the python colab runtime to cause a runtime warning due to divide by zero error for incalculably small edges. In subsequent phases, this uncomputed vertex creates non-alphanumeric value(nan).

In this paper, the main contributions are:

i) An improved scale dependant umbrella mesh denoising algorithm (ISDUMD) is proposed that corrects the SDU algorithm up to 4.21% using the Bayesian Averaging Method (BAM) [13].
ii) BAM is used to determine the average of a distribution from a predetermined average. The constant 'c' in the BAM is experimentally determined at 0.001.
iii) The constant c and BAM-mean are added to the vertex calculations which removes the runtime error for the subsequent stages. The result shows an overall 4.21% improvement of the proposed algorithm over the SDU algorithm

2 Smoothing Techniques (Surface Fairing)

2.1 Laplacian Smoothing

The theory behind Laplacian smoothing is similar to image blurring [14] where one vertex is averaged over its neighbourhood vertices. The operator is Laplace-Beltrami operator [15]. In Eq. 1 ngbi is the neighbourhood set of vertex i. Laplacian smoothing causes the image to shrink and this can be slowed by the λ constant as the weight factor on the displacement vector [16].

2.2 HC-Algorithm

HC-algorithm (Humphery's class) [9] is an improved Laplacian method where the shrunken vertex is pushed back to a relative position such that the new location is depend on the difference of displacement around the neighbourhood from the original position [1] as shown in Eq. 3.

2.3 Taubin's Signal Processing Approach

The basic idea of Taubin's method is similar to HC-algorithm, but in this approach two balancing weights are used λ and μ. The λ constant causes the mesh shrinkage and μ constant de-shrinks the mesh because it holds a negative value. The value of λ is taken as 0.67 and the value for μ is -0.33.

2.4 Mean Curvature Flow (MCF)

Desburn et al. [11] proposed the mean curvature flow to approximate the Laplacian. The basic idea was to calculate the sum of the opposite cotangent of the common neighbours and use it as a weight factor. The curvature flow only allows for the vertex to move along the normal direction only limiting any tangential movement at the current vertex of observation. The curvature normal of a vertex is given as shown in Eq. 4, where A is the area covered around the central vertex. The - ve sign in Eq. 4 is to counter the volume shrinkage which happens while smoothing.

2.5 Scale Dependent Umbrella (SDU)

The SDU algorithm is based on the Laplacian operator but the effect of each vertex depends on the edge length. Shorter the distance of a vertex from the central vertex, more is the influence and stronger pull towards that neighbour.

3 Related Work

As the mesh structure of any object highly resembles a topology [17], the field of topology optimization (TO) also relates to computing efficient surface structure [18]. Additive manufacturing (AM) techniques [19] adds materials within a particular region on top of an existing object to create the final output. This technique allows high precision material construction as compared to the traditional manner of construction, where extra materials are removed from the top layer of an object by means of carving, shaping, milling, etc. [1]. AM and TO are combined [20, 21] to achieve improved performance The denoising of the external surfaces is inspired by techniques in image processing [22, 23]. Lee et al. [24] proposed a feature-preserving mesh denoising algorithm. The algorithm is a two-stage process. In the first stage, the surface normal is selected and in the second, normals are summed for least square error (LSE) in the update of the new vertex position. Anisotropic diffusion [25] introduces intra region smoothing as compared to inter-region smoothing. The experiment is like varying Gaussian filters applied to a signal at different scales [26]. Robust estimation [27] is based on the fact that for smooth surfaces, the normal vary smoothly. The surface is then formulated as a level-set of volumes and is expected to fit the parameters solved from partial differential equations (PDEs) and in the process to do so the normal is predefined. Bilateral filtering [28] is a noniterative and local process. It combines region intensity based on geometric proximity and photometric similarity, giving preference to closer values. The methods described in [29–31] are based on functional parametrization and control point movement. These methods are based on signal processing approach and minimization of an energy function such as the squared magnitude of the curvature and estimation of function coefficients. Structure optimization is not limited to medical images but expands to wide areas in aerospace [32], automotive [33], and biomedicine [34]. TO is about minimizing a fitness function which can either be the structure or volume reduction and maximizing one global value such as stiffness. The boundary condition associated with TO problems must be known beforehand, such as the information of the number of holes, texture information, initial and final volume, and surface area [35]. Numerous TO optimization techniques are found in the literature such as solid isotropic material with penalization (SIMP) [36]. Evolutionary structural optimization method (ESO) [37] and bi-directional ESO (BESO) [38]. In [39] individual-level activation measurements in brain fMRI in unreliable and hence group-level analyses are considered, using the Bayesian general linear model (GLM). In the paper [40] prior $\pi(\theta)$ is assumed for Bayesian evidence measurement as an average of the likelihood. Spencer et al. [41] uses prior brain study to include expected behaviour for smoothing and sensitivity error corrections. Geng et al. [42] propose an ensemble method that uses Bayesian extreme learning machines (BELM) to train with historical scans of multiple objects for the correction of acquired point cloud data.

4 Proposed Work

The Bayesian averaging method [13] as shown in Eq. 5 is estimating the mean using apriori information. Here, to find the mean of the vertex, it is assumed that the mean is already known from previous models, and constant c is experimentally determined to be 0.001. The value of m is calculated from 5 different models consisting of 2 female and 3 male whole brain MR from the dataset UPENN-GBM [43]. In line number 10 of the proposed Algorithm (see Sect. 9), the division by zero runtime operation is handled properly after the inclusion of the proposed method, rest of the algorithm is same as SDU. Procedure get mean prepares a mean model and get Bayesian average calculates the Bayesian mean. The block diagram of the model is shown in Fig. 1.

5 Results and Discussion

From Table 1 it can be seen that Taubin's method attained acceptable model reconstruction after 5 iterations, but due to expansion of the shrinking model, the volume and surface area 75.13 mm 3 and 123.22 mm 2 respectively is highest amongst all methods. It is also seen that the total change is also the highest amongst all algorithms at 2258 mm. The volume of MCF is closest to the original volume at 52.25 mm 3. The number of iterations taken by MCF for the optimum model smoothing is 30 and the time taken in seconds is 650, which is highest amongst all algorithms. The proposed (SDU + BAM) method is seen to improve the the SDU algorithm generated model volume by $\approx 2\%$ and surface area by $\approx 1.3\%$ in 16.67% less number of iterations. Table 4 is the change in surface volume measured from Eq. 7. From (Fig. 3(b)) it is seen that the proposed model follows the Laplacian model (Refer Table 3) due to the averaging step which is close to the Laplacian technique. The SDU algorithm after each itearation smoothens the vertex, thus reducing edge lengths, it stops to respond after iteration 20, when no longer edges are numerically greater than 0. (Fig. 3(a)) shows that the volume deviation of the SDU is lowered after iteration 20. From Fig. 4 it is seen that the proposed (SDU + BAM) model has 4.21% increased accuracy from the noise model. It is calculated by subtracting the noisy SSIM from the smoothed SSIM $0.71 - 0.6813 / 0.6813 \times 100 = 4.21\%$(Refer Table 2). All experiments were performed on 0.6813 Google Colab developing environment. For Comparison and competent results in Table 3 and Table 4 the noise was reduced and SSIM was increased to 0.8906 and MSE was reduced to 128.2186. Refer Fig. 7 for the error in surface reconstruction. It can be seen that the proposed method is improved over the existing SDU algorithm. The time complexity of the proposed algorithm is $O(p + V)$, where p is number of models used in mean calculation and V is number of vertices in the mean model (Fig. 5).

6 Figures

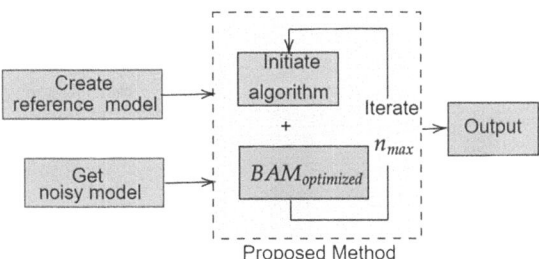

Fig. 1. Block diagram of the proposed model

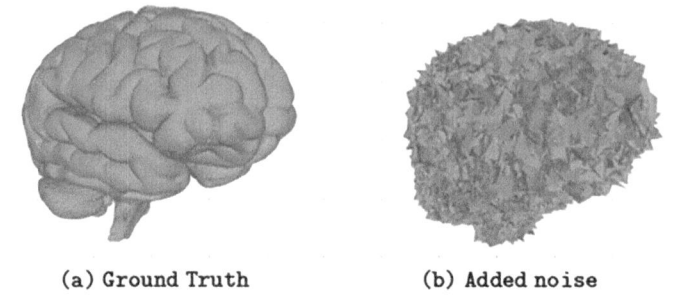

(a) Ground Truth **(b) Added noise**

Fig. 2. (a) Brain model in ground truth (b) Brain model with 33.217 dB noise

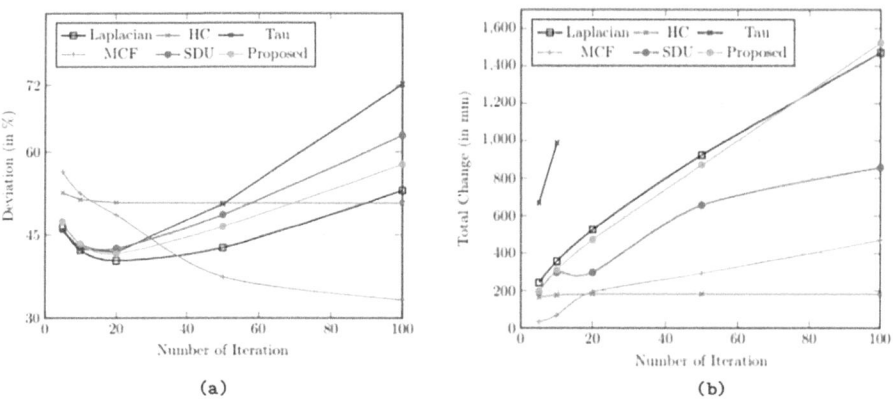

Fig. 3. (a) % change in deviation (b) change in volume

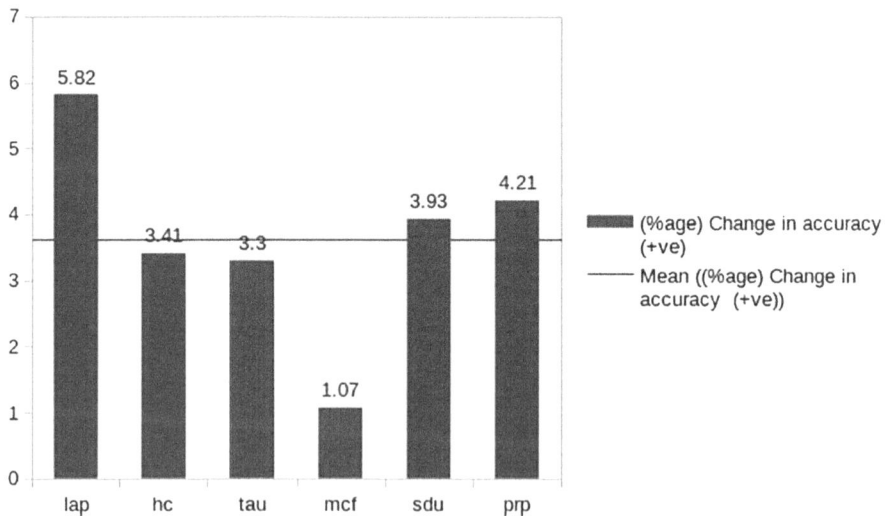

Fig. 4. % change in accuracy

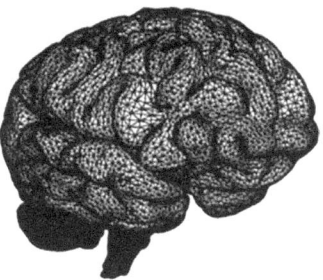

Fig. 5. Average vertex locations

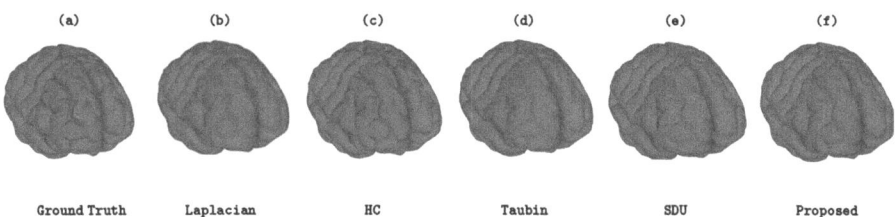

Fig. 6. (a) Ground truth (b) Laplacian (c) HC (d) Taubin (e) SDU (f) Proposed. (b-f) are smoother surface of noisy input generated by each algorithm after 10 iterations.

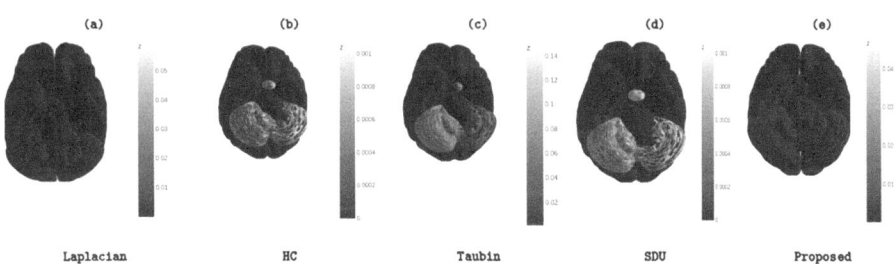

Fig. 7. Error map in smoothed brain structure after 10 iterations for the algorithms (a) Laplacian (b) HC (c) Taubin (d) SDU (e) Proposed

7 Tables

Table 1. Comparison of denoising algorithms for smoothing a brain model

Method	Volume (mm^3)	Surface (mm^2)	Time (s)	Number of iterations	Total change (mm)
Original	53.57	108.85	-	-	-
Laplacian	49.45	94.40	140	15	1278
HC	52.92	102.36	120	8	1268
Taubin	75.13	123.22	110	5	2258
MCF	52.25	103.17	650	30	1295
SDU	49.54	95.91	280	12	1278
Proposed (SDU + BAM)	50.53	97.18	260	10	1292

Table 2. Comparison of SSIM and MSE after smoothing a 33.217 db PSNR random noise brain model

Method	SSIM	MSE
Ground Truth (Fig. 2a)	0.6813	539.8907
Laplacian (Fig. 6b)	0.721	373.059
HC (Fig. 6c)	0.7046	1439.996
Taubin (Fig. 6d)	0.7038	1138.5714
MCF	0.6886	874.198
SDU (Fig. 6e)	0.7081	1074.057
Proposed (SDU + BAM) (Fig. 6f)	0.7100	1078.541

Table 3. Comparison of denoising algorithms for the total change (mm)

Number of iterations	Algorithms					
	Laplacian	HC	Taubin	MCF	SDU	Proposed (SDU + BAM)
5	242	163	669	32	192	195
10	356	176	988	68	297	308
20	527	181		193	297	473
50	924	181		292	659	871
100	1471	181		471	857	1524

Table 4. Comparison of denoising algorithms for the total deviation (%)

Number of iterations	Algorithms					
	Laplacian	HC	Taubin	MCF	SDU	Proposed (SDU + BAM)
5	46.24	52.6	45.75	56.4	47.3	47.3
10	42.22	51.4	42.47	52.5	43.4	43.4
20	40.33	50.9	41.87	48.6	42.6	41.6
50	42.7	50.8	50.58	37.4	48.65	46.5
100	53.04	50.8	72.23	33.3	62.96	57.75

8 Equations

$$newcordinate = \frac{1}{size(ngb_i)} \sum_{j \in ngb_i} cordinate_j \qquad (1)$$

$$shrink_j = \alpha \cdot original_j + (1-\alpha) \cdot cordinate_j, \alpha \in [0,1] \qquad (2)$$

$$difference_i = new\,cordinate_i - shrink_i \qquad (3)$$

$$relative_i = \beta \cdot differnece_i + \frac{1-\beta}{size(ngb_i)} \sum_{j \in ngb_i} \beta \in [0,1]$$

$$-\overline{k}n = \frac{1}{4A} \sum_{j \in ngb_i} (\cot \alpha_j + \cot \beta_j)(cordinate_j - cordinate_i) \qquad (4)$$

$$\overline{x} = \frac{cm + \sum_{i=1}^{n} x_j}{c+n} \qquad (5)$$

$$total\,change = \sum_{i \in vertices} change_i \qquad (6)$$

$$deviation = \left(\frac{surface\,area_{model}}{surface\,area_{sphere}} - 1 \right) \times 100 \qquad (7)$$

9 Algorithm

Procedure get_mean(Models)
    While i in Models do
        n is size(Models)
        if n >0 then
            m is average coordinates
        end if
    end while
    return m
end procedure

Procedure get_Bayesian_average(Models)
    $c \in [0,1]$
    m is get_mean(Models)
    while i is vertices do
        n is size(ngb(i))
        if n>0 then
$$BMA = \frac{cm + \sum_{i=1}^{n} x_j}{c+n}$$
        End if
    End while
    Return BMA

End Procedure

Proposed Algorithm: SDU + BAM
c is 0.001
$\acute{x}$ is get_Bayesian_average(Models)
While iter <= max do
    While i is vertices do
        n is size(ngb(i)) if n >0
        while j $\in$ ngb(i) do
            get difference
            get shrink
        end while
        new coordinate= cordniate + difference/shrink
    end while
end while

10 Conclusion and Future Work

Amongst all the five different methods implemented in this case, the Laplacian method is the most suitable due to its simple algorithm, fast running time and no possibility of division by 0 error. As SDU computes the area, truncating the decimal causes a negligible area. The proposed method is able to improve the SDU algorithm in situations where the SDU raises a division by 0 error when it is constrained with precision up to 2 decimal places. In the experimental model the added noise is random and deliberately made high to access the smoothing metrics better. The possible outcomes for lower and other types of noises will be studied in the future along with test cases consisting of other types of human organs.

Disclosure of Interests. The authors have no competing interests to declare that are relevant to the content of this article.

References

1. Bacciaglia, A., Ceruti, A., Liverani, A.: Surface smoothing for topological optimized 3D models. Struct. Multi. Optim. **64**(6), 3453–3472 (2021)
2. Rublee, E., et al.: Orb: An eff. Alt. to sift or surf. In: 2011 International Conference on CV, pp. 2564–2571. IEEE (2011)
3. Rublee, E., Rabaud, V., Konolige, K., Bradski, G.: ORB: An efficient alternative to SIFT or SURF. In: 2011 International Conference on Computer Vision, pp. 2564–2571. IEEE (2021)
4. Szegedy, C., Ioffe, S., Vanhoucke, V., Alemi, A.A.: Inception-v4, inception-resnet and the impact of residual connections on learning. In: Thirty-first AAAI Conference on Artificial Intelligence (2017)
5. Li, J., et al.: The 3d reconstruction of a digital model for irregular gangue blocks and its application in pfc numerical simulation. Eng. Comput. 1–11(2021)
6. Kohlberger, T., Singh, V., Alvino, C., Bahlmann, C., Grady, L.: Evaluating segmentation error without ground truth. In: International Conference on Medical Image Computing and Computer-Assisted Intervention, pp. 528–536.Springer (2012)
7. Lorensen, W.E., Cline, H.E.: Marching cubes: a high resolution 3d surface construction algorithm. ACM Siggraph Comput. Graph. **21**(4), 163–169 (1987)
8. Sorkine, O.: Laplacian mesh processing. Eurographics (State of the Art Reports) **4** (2005)
9. Vollmer, J., Mencl, R., Mueller, H.: Improved laplacian smoothing of noisy surface meshes. In: Computer Graphics Forum, vol. 18, pp. 131–138. Wiley Online Library (1999)
10. Taubin, G.: A signal processing approach to fair surface design. In: Proceedings of the 22nd Annual Conference on Computer Graphics and Interactive Techniques, pp. 351–358 (1995)
11. Desbrun, M., Meyer, M., Schröder, P., Barr, A.H.: Implicit fairing of irregular meshes using diffusion and curvature flow. In: Proceedings of the 26th Annual Conference on Computer Graphics and Interactive Techniques, pp. 317–324 (1999)
12. Fujiwara, K.: Eigenvalues of laplacians on a closed riemannian manifold and its nets. Proc. Am. Math. Soc. **123**(8), 2585–2594 (1995)
13. Raftery, A.E., Madigan, D., Hoeting, J.A.: Bayesian model averaging for linear regression models. J. Am. Stat. Assoc. **92**(437), 179–191 (1997)
14. Wang, D.C., Vagnucci, A.H., Li, C.C.: Digital image enhancement: a survey. Comput. Vis. Graph. Image Process. **24**(3), 363–381 (1983)
15. Xu, G.: Discrete laplace–beltrami operators and their convergence. CAGD **21**(8), 767–784 (2004)
16. Bobenko, A.I., Springborn, B.A.: A discrete laplace–beltrami operator for simplicial surfaces. Discret. Comput. Geom. **38**(4), 740–756 (2007)
17. Li, H., et al.: Appl. Math. Model. **101**, 276–308 (2022)
18. Bendsoe, M.P., Sigmund, O.: Topology optimization: theory, methods, and applications. Springer Science & Business Media (2013)
19. Gao, W., et al.: The status, challenges, and future of additive manufacturing in engineering. Comput. Aided Des. **69**, 65–89 (2015)
20. Gaynor, A.T., Meisel, N.A., Williams, C.B., Guest, J.K.: J. Manufact. Sci. Eng. **136**(6) (2014)

21. Rezaie, R., Badrossamay, M., Ghaie, A., Moosavi, H.: Topology optimization for fused deposition modeling process. Procedia Cirp **6**, 521–526 (2013)
22. Buades, A., Coll, B., Morel, J.-M.: A review of image denoising algorithms, with a new one. Multiscale Model. Simul. **4**(2), 490–530 (2005)
23. Zhang, M., Gunturk, B.K.: Multiresolution bilateral filtering for image denoising. IEEE Trans. Image Process. **17**(12), 2324–2333 (2008)
24. Lee, K.W., Wang, W.P.: Feature-preserving mesh denoising via bilateral normal filtering. In: Ninth International Conference on Computer Aided Design and Computer Graphics (CAD-CG'05), p. 6. IEEE (2005)
25. Perona, P., Malik, J.: Scale-space and edge detection using anisotropic diffusion. IEEE Trans. Pattern Anal. Mach. Intell. **12**(7), 629–639 (1990)
26. Witkin, A.: Scale space filtering. in int. joint conference on artificial intelligence (karlsruhe, germany) (1983)
27. Tasdizen, T., Whitaker, R., Burchard, P., Osher, S.: Geometric surface processing via normal maps. ACM Trans. Graph. (TOG) **22**(4), 1012–1033 (2003)
28. Tomasi, C., Manduchi, R.: Bilateral filtering for gray and color images. In: Sixth International Conference on Computer Vision (IEEE Cat. No. 98CH36271), pp. 839–846. IEEE (1998)
29. Moreton, H.P., Séquin, C.H.: Functional optimization for fair surface design. ACM SIGGRAPH Comput. Graph. **26**(2), 167–176 (1992)
30. Welch, W., Witkin, A.: Variational surface modeling. ACM SIGGRAPH Comput. Graph. **26**(2), 157–166 (1992)
31. Guskov, I., Sweldens, W., Schröder, P.: Proceedings of the 26th Annual Conference on Computer Graphics and Interactive Techniques, pp. 325–334 (1999)
32. Wong, J., Ryan, L., Kim, I.: Struct. Multidiscip. Optim. **57**(3), 1357–1375 (2018)
33. Mantovani, S., Barbieri, S.G., Giacopini, M., Croce, A., Sola, A., Bassoli, E.: Proceedings of the Institution of Mechanical Engineers. Part B: J. Eng. Manuf. **235**(3), 555–567 (2021)
34. Machado, G., Trabucho, L.: Some results in topology optimization applied to biomechanics. Comput. Struct. **82**(17–19), 1389–1397 (2004)
35. Sigmund, O.: On the design of compliant mechanisms using topology optimization. J. Struct. Mech. **25**(4), 493–524 (1997)
36. Bendsøe, M.P.: Optimal shape design as a material distribution problem. Struct. Optim. **1**(4), 193–202 (1989)
37. Xie, Y., Steven, G.: Evolutionary structural optimization for dynamic problems. Comput. Struct. **58**(6), 1067–1073 (1996)
38. Li, Q., Steven, G., Xie, Y.: A simple checkerboard suppression algorithm for evolutionary structural optimization. Struct. Multidiscip. Optim. **22**(3), 230–239 (2001)
39. Spencer, D., Yue, Y.R., Bolin, D., Ryan, S., Mejia, A.F.: Spatial bayesian glm on the cortical surface produces reliable task activations in individuals and groups. Neuroimage **249**, 118908 (2022)
40. Koo, H., Keeley, R.E., Shafieloo, A., L'Huillier, B.: J. Cosmol. Astropart. Phys. **2022**(03), 047 (2022)
41. Spencer, D., Bolin, D., Nebel, M.B., Mejia, A.: Fast Bayesian estimation of brain activation with cortical surface and subcortical fMRI data using EM (2022). arXiv preprint arXiv:2203.00053
42. Geng, Z., Sabbaghi, A., Bidanda, B.: Automated variance modeling for three dimensional point cloud data via bayesian neural networks. IISE Trans. (just-accepted), 1–27 (2022)
43. Bakas, S., et al.: The university of pennsylvania glioblastoma (UPenn-GBM) cohort: advanced MRI, clinical, genomics, & radiomics. Sci. Data **9**(1), 453 (2022)
44. Gostler, A. Processing medical surface meshes for 3d printing. Master's thesis, Faculty of Informatics, Vienna University of Technology (2016)
45. Hore, A., Ziou, D. Image Quality Metrics: PSNR vs. SSIM. In: 2010 20th International Conference on Pattern Recognition, pp. 2366–2369. IEEE (2010)

Traumatic Condition Assessment and Monitoring Through Retinal Fundus Image

Gaurav Sharma[1], Maninder Singh[2(✉)], Basant Kumar[2], K. M. Soni[1], and Deepak Agrawal[3]

[1] Amity Institute of Information Technology, Amity University, Noida 201313, India
[2] Electronics and Communication Engineering Department, Motilal Nehru National Institute of Technology Allahabad, Prayagraj 211004, India
maninder.2018rel07@mnnit.ac.in
[3] All India Institute of Medical Sciences, JPNATC, New Delhi 110029, India

Abstract. The paper presents a segmentation method of the artery and vein in the fundus retinal image using the deep learning architecture U-Net. In the segmentation of the artery and vein, the architecture is hyper tuned using the optimizers at a learning rate of 0.001 and 0.01. The segmentation of artery and vein is performed on the retinal fundus imaging, that can be helpful for the early assessment of traumatic conditions in patients' diagnosis with the head injury. The traumatic conditions are related to the intracranial pressure (ICP) which is correlated with artery-vein diameter, optic disc cup ratio, and retinal tortuosity. It has been concluded that these parameters containing information for multiple measures with and without papilledema symptoms can be a breakthrough for the traumatic disorder. The performance of the segmented artery and vein is evaluated for three different optimizers by evaluating the optimal accuracy, sensitivity and specificity. The optimal accuracy for the NADAM optimizer at a learning rate of 0.001 and batch size of 8 is 93.70%. Further, sensitivity and specificity were computed for the DRIVE database which found to be 92.35 and 93.41 respectively.

Keywords: Intracranial Pressure · Arteriovenous Ratio · Cup to Disc Ratio · Retinal Tortuosity

1 Introduction

Trauma condition can be chronicled as a sudden event happening in individual life as physically or threatening that harms the individual and has an adverse effect. These trauma conditions are classified depending on the type of injury; it varies from primary to secondary type and is classified as injury related to cerebral edema, contusions, intracranial hemorrhage, hematoma, and increased intracranial pressure (ICP) [1][2]. ICP disorders can occur for various reasons, such as mass lesions in the brain, an increase in cerebrospinal fluid (CSF), and other pathological processes [3]. Due to these disorders, ICP arises, and in such situations monitoring and its measurement are compulsory

---

G. Sharma, M. Singh, B. Kumar, K.M. Soni, D. Agrawa—Contributed equally to this work.

and are challenging tasks in clinical practice. The causes of traumatic situations and their diagnostic behavior are demonstrated in Fig. 1. The critical diagnostic parameters indicating trauma conditions are cerebrospinal fluid (CSF), cerebral perfusion pressure (CPP) and raised intracranial pressure (ICP). The CSF formation mathematical model [4][5] has been developed in the literature by explaining the various factors to maintain the stable state of ICP. In the central nervous system (CNS), the CSF consists of extra-cellular fluid, CSF as a fluid takes care of the spinal cord and the brain protecting them from injury. The other important aspect of measuring intracranial pressure is calculating cerebral perfusion pressure (CPP) in brain-injured patients. The parameter cerebral perfusion pressure can be considered to be an optimizing pressure in patients suffering from traumatic injury. The cerebral perfusion pressure monitoring will help in achieving the desired outcome in selecting an optimal value for the intracranial pressure.

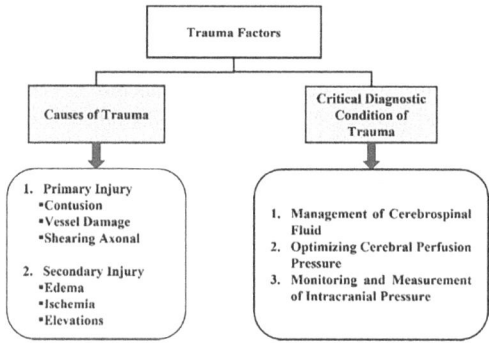

Fig. 1. Traumatic situations and their diagnostic behaviour.

Monitoring the intracranial pressure in neuro-intensive care required a critically ill patient suffering from traumatic brain injury, space-occupying lesions, hematoma, and hemorrhage. The indirect measurement of ICP by a non-invasive method such as lumbar puncture in concurrence with an assessment of resistance to cerebrospinal fluid outflow is treated as a clinical routine for diagnostics of chronic health. Although, it is evident from the Monro-Kellie theory [6] that in the skull, the volume of the main contents, such as CSF and brain parenchyma, along with brain tissue, needs to be in proportion of approximately 1700 ml. The changes in any of the contents need to be compensated by the other contents in the skull, if in any condition, the contents in the skull are not compensated, then the intracranial pressure (ICP) increases and is exhausted at some point. In the skull contents, cerebrospinal fluid's main components are a major fluid used in maintaining the level and keeping ICP stable. Figure 2 illustrates all three conditions when due to displacement, the mass increases and due to that there is a change in composition and affecting the ICP. Retinal fundus imaging can be used to measure the intracranial pressure for possible early diagnosis and treatment using the various methods for different parameters. The main objective of the proposed research work is to discuss various challenges related to retinal fundus imaging role in measuring and monitoring traumatic conditions in the early stages. The abnormalities in the optic disc, retinal tortuosity, and arteriole ventriole measurement, have not been studied well is discussed.

Further, the segmentation of the artery and vein in fundus retinal image using the deep learning architecture is performed and performance evaluation of the segmented vessels is done. Further, the main contribution of our work can be summarized as follows:

1. An automated method is presented for the segmentation of artery vein in retinal fundus imaging, the NADAM optimizer achieved the better accuracy in segmenting the vessels.
2. The role of artery vein, optic cup to disc and retinal tortuosity is discussed that can play major role in early diagnosis and continuous monitoring of traumatic patients.

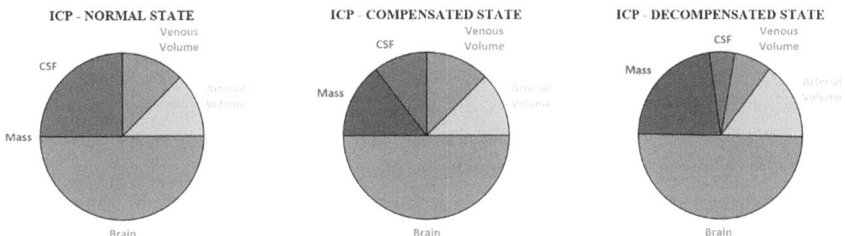

Fig. 2. Monro-Kellie composition affecting the ICP

2 Literature Survey

The literature data is related to the retinal fundus imaging, which plays a vital role in diagnosing and treating the traumatic condition of the patients. The traumatic behaviour in retinopathy generally occurs due to the complicated injury. Later, these results in poor visual outcomes in patients, resulting in the severe evaluation and decision-making in such conditions. The ICP measures the traumatic disorder with the help of invasive measurement or non-invasive measurement, which will be helpful in indicating the state of the patient by the ophthalmologist. The various ophthalmologists include information of the optic disc after the measurement in diagnosis of trauma condition. The information in the optic disc may be a signal for the presence of papilledema, which is indicative of ICP. In the Monro Kellie's doctrine theory, the lesion that occupies space in the brain, leads to intracranial hypertension and can cause the formation of papilledema, which refers to swelling of the optic disc. However, vision loss occurs due to other pathological reasons such as retinal detachments, haemorrhage, or choroidal folds.

Digre et al. [7] compared a case study for intracranial hypertension in patients suffering from papilledema condition and without papilledema. It stated the possibility that intracranial hypertension can occur in the absence of papilledema, and it should be considered a clinical condition for visual loss. Kashif et al. [8] described the model for the ICP estimation, it includes main cerebrovascular compartments with variables such as cerebral blood flow (CBF), arterial blood pressure (ABP), and ICP. The non-invasive measurements of 45 patients are performed by including recording ABP, CBF, and invasive ICP waveforms. Hamill et al. [9] discussed the role of the cup to disc ratio (CDR) in idiopathic intracranial hypertension (IIH) with papilledema symptoms and without papilledema. Interestingly, small CDR in patients with intracranial hypertension without papilledema may be useful for comparing the findings with CDR in patients with intracranial hypertension. Saba et al. [10] distinguish the papilledema using deep learning U-NET and Dense Net architecture and grading of papilledema performed by the vasculature structure. Andersen et al. [11] proposed a correlation between the ICP and artery-vein (A/V) ratio. The dataset includes 24 patients that are suffering from normal pressure hydrocephalus (NPH) and ventriculoperitoneal (VP) shunt dysfunction. Further, the correlation between the A/V ratio and ICP was obtained and used as a non-invasive method to estimate the traumatic condition. Ghate et al. [12] experimented on the pig model and concluded that ICP changes occur with the changes in the retinal vein diameter, and the information can be helpful in the traumatic condition. Further, the Dashtbozorg et al. [13] have used a graph-based approach to classify the artery and vein using fundus imaging. The network is drawn as an undirected graph which is divided into several subgraphs. The method uses Inspire, Drive and Vicavr databases to evaluate the network's accuracy values. Martinez-Perez et al. [14] have extracted the vessel using derivative features and two-stage region from red-free and fluorescein photographs. Estrada et al. [15] classified the artery vein by topology-based method. In exploring the framework, the domain-specific features are used to construct the likelihood model and the possible solutions in classifying the vessels. The model's performance is evaluated on WIDE, AV-Drive and CT-Drive datasets. Xu et al. [16] have distinguished the artery vein on Drive database, using the intra image regularization and inter subject normalization by the texture features. Guo et al. [17] have identified the artery vein with the help of a convolutional neural network (CNN) and reinforcement sample learning scheme. The performance of the model has been evaluated by computing the accuracy for the segmentation of the artery and vein on Drive and Stare databases. Kang et al. [18] have explored the attention weighted fusion approach to segment artery vein and further vascular structure reconstruction algorithm has improved the model's performance for the three datasets, namely Drive, LES-AV and WIDE.

3 Measurement

The fundus camera imaging can be viewed from various angles depending on the experienced ophthalmologist and different software for visualizing a retinal image. The ophthalmologist uses prior knowledge to correctly measure arterioles and venules, optic CDR, tortuosity index, and other fundus image abnormalities. In Fig. 3, the schematic diagram of the ICP assessment is shown.

3.1 Arteries and Veins Measurement

The measurement of retinal arteries and veins diameters was to analyze the association with hypertension to predict ICP. Initially, Bailliart [19] stated that a retinal blood vessel has a relation to the ocular pressure and measures with the help of an ophthalmodynamometer, but later various digital measuring methods were used for the measurement of blood vessel diameter. Firsching [20] reported the retinal outflow pressure with the

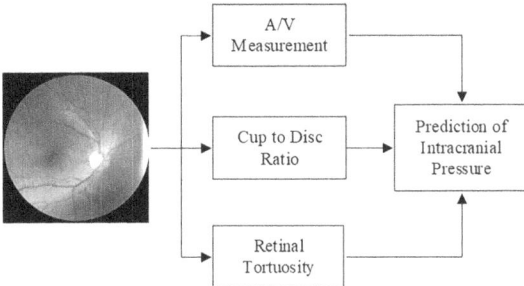

Fig. 3. The schematic diagram for the assessment of ICP

ICP and found that the reduced arteriole and venule diameter ratio is associated with the optic disc swelling. In elevated cerebrospinal fluid, intracranial hypertension abnormalities are proportional to the retinal arterial-vein diameter and blood pressure. The spontaneous retinal venous pulsation association in the patients with high ICP discussed by Wong [21], the SRVP is caused near the optic disk and further correlated the relation to the cerebrospinal fluid. In another study, Linda [22] uses infrared recording to assess venous pulsation and ICP; additionally, the interpretation of fundus images requires experienced ophthalmologists to identify SVP. Using the deep learning architecture, some literature finds the characteristics of these vessel diameters. In adolescent children, Yuan [23] examined that the blood pressure can be correlated to the blood vessel diameter and reported that excessive blood pressure was connected with narrower arterioles and has no association with retinal venules. These studies' investigation suggests that retinal vessel diameter will need to be explored with respect to the changes in blood pressure, CSF, and SVP to predict the ICP.

In a clinical, the early prediction of trauma conditions is a challenge for the researcher to predict the behavior of the ICP concerning the retina vessels. The retina vessel measurement can be subdivided into parts, with the primary objective of classifying artery and vein. The vessel segments were performed to extract the artery and vein information based on color, features, and properties. The most publicly available datasets, such as DRIVE and STARE, can be used to segment vessels with respect to other available datasets and measure the performance of the proposed method. Table 1 gives the publicly available dataset detail.

Secondly, after the classification of vessels, its diameter measurement is of importance where the ratio calculated for correlating with the ICP in hypertension. In correlation large sample size is needed in associating the A/V ratio with hypertension patients with ICP. Previously, an ophthalmologist measured the diameter at the radii of 0.5 to 1 from the optic Disc for the A/V ratio. An automated method uses the Euclidean distance relation for the diameter measurement. The length of the shortest path determined the artery and vein diameters through the centerline pixels inside the vessel region. Further, the A/V ratio is calculated by the central artery equivalent and the central venular equivalent ratio [24].

$$CAE = \sqrt{0.87 W_{sa} + 1.01 W_{la} - 0.22 W_{sa} W_{lb} - 10.76} \quad (1)$$

Table 1. Publicly available dataset for artery-vein segmentation

Database	Image
RITE (Retinal Images vessel Tree Extraction)	40
DRIVE: Digital Retinal Images for Vessel Extraction	40
INSPIRE-AVR (Iowa Normative Set for Processing Images of the Retina)	40
High-Resolution Fundus (HRF)	45
STARE (Structured Analysis of the Retina)	50
LES-AV dataset	22

$$CVE = \sqrt{0.72W_{sv}^2 + 0.91W_{lv}^2 + 450.05} \quad (2)$$

where,

W_{sa} = width of small arteriole; W_{sa} = width of small arteriole;
W_{sv} = width of small venule; W_{lv} = width of large venule

Further, it can be concluded that using deep learning and machine learning modules, the segmentation of arteries and veins is a primary objective in classifying the vessels. Figure 4 shows the extracted artery vein where the artery is indicated by the red color and the vein by the blue color. A secondary aim A/V ratio measurement follows it. In the proposed work the deep learning architecture is applied to segment the artery-vein using the retinal fundus is explained below.

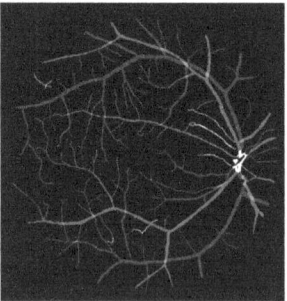

Fig. 4. Artery-Vein extraction using fundus image

Segmentation of Artery-Vein Using Deep Network In the proposed work, the database is trained on the deep learning architecture. In training the architecture, several augmentation strategies are been applied. The augmentation includes scaling for a scale factor of 0.2, shifting at 0.1 and rotation at an angle of 10 degrees. The deep learning model is trained and tested to obtain a segmented image of a retinal fundus image. Table 2 demonstrates the encoder decoder architecture of U-net which is used for the artery vein segmentation. The architecture has a convolutional layer which is followed by the max pooling layer in the encoder path, the activation function ReLU is defined for each layer.

The decoder path uses a concatenation operation followed by the convolutional layer. Each layer uses the ReLU activation function except for the last layer, where the sigmoid activation function is used. The function binary cross entropy quantifies the loss of the artery vein segmentation. In training the network, several optimizers are chosen to optimize the model for a learning rate of 0.001 and 0.01. Initially, the learning rate is set at 0.01 and then varies to 0.001 for batch sizes 4 and 8. The training of the network is hyper-tuned to obtain the appropriate accuracy. The performance of the artery vein segmentation and its classification has been evaluated.

Table 2. Architecture for Artery vein performed on Drive Database

Layer	Output Size	Filter Size	Stride
Inputs	576 × 576 × 3	3 × 3	1 × 1
Conv 1	576 × 576 × 32	3 × 3	1 × 1
Conv 2	576 × 576 × 32	3 × 3	1 × 1
Max Pool 1	288 × 288 × 32	3 × 3	1 × 1
Conv 3	288 × 288 × 64	3 × 3	1 × 1
Conv 4	288 × 288 × 64	3 × 3	1 × 1
Max Pool 2	144 × 144 × 64	3 × 3	1 × 1
Conv 5	144 × 144 × 128	3 × 3	1 × 1
Conv 6	144 × 144 × 128	3 × 3	1 × 1
Max Pool 3	72 × 72 × 128	3 × 3	1 × 1
Conv 7	72 × 72 × 256	3 × 3	1 × 1
Conv 8	72 × 72 × 256	3 × 3	1 × 1
Max Pool 4	36 × 36 × 256	3 × 3	1 × 1
Conv 9	36 × 36 × 512	3 × 3	1 × 1
Conv 10	36 × 36 × 512	3 × 3	1 × 1
Up Sampling 1	72 × 72 × 512	2 × 2	2 × 2
Conv 11	72 × 72 × 256	3 × 3	1 × 1
Conv 12	72 × 72 × 256	3 × 3	1 × 1
Up Sampling 2	144 × 144 × 256	2 × 2	2 × 2
Conv 13	144 × 144 × 128	3 × 3	1 × 1
Conv 14	144 × 144 × 128	3 × 3	1 × 1
Up Sampling 3	288 × 288 × 128	2 × 2	2 × 2
Conv 15	288 × 288 × 64	3 × 3	1 × 1

(*continued*)

Table 2. (continued)

Layer	Output Size	Filter Size	Stride
Conv 16	288 × 288 × 64	3 × 3	1 × 1
Up Sampling 4	576 × 576 × 64	2 × 2	2 × 2
Conv 17	576 × 576 × 32	3 × 3	1 × 1
Conv 18	576 × 576 × 32	3 × 3	1 × 1
Output	576 × 576 × 1	1 × 1	1 × 1

3.2 Cup to Disc Ratio Measurement

The optic cup to disc ratio (CDR) is the diameter of cup C divided by the diameter of disc D in the retinal. Figure 5 shows the disc and cup in a fundus image. A limited study has been done on the optic CDR in association with ICP. The optic CDR ratio study was performed on patients suffering from intracranial hypertension where vision loss is concerned. It correlated with the small optic CDR found in such a population [25]. In the diagnosis of the optic CDR in children suffering from intracranial hypertension [26], it is similar that most of the cups are generally absent or small in such cases of the optic disc. Further, in a patient suffering from venous sinus thrombosis [27], there is an optic cup loss with the diagnosis of papilledema and intracranial hypertension increased.

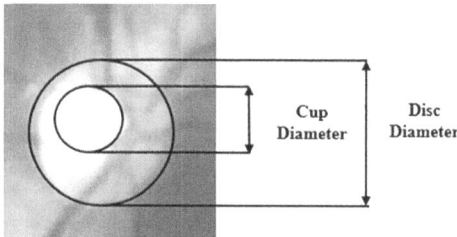

Fig. 5. Cup to disc representation in the fundus image

The measurement of optic CDR using a color fundus image can be accomplished by segmenting the optic cup and optic disc. The optic cup is more visible and can be distinguished easily in the green channel, and the optic disc is a brighter region and can be distinguished easily in the red channel image. CDR measurement consists of many stages: area of interest extraction, pre-processing, extraction of diagnostic parameters based on feature extraction, and classification. ROI extraction is performed to extract the region around the optic disc instead of the complete image, significantly reducing the detection's computational complexity and computation time. Pre-processing of the fundus image used to remove noise and increase the contrast. The feature extraction of the CDR uses various methods such as Circular Hough Transform, K-means clustering, and CNN. Further, the diagnostic parameters, namely CDR, are calculated, which help to decide the correlation with ICP in a traumatic condition.

3.3 Retinal Tortuosity

The retina vasculature sometimes appears in a non-smooth way as it changes its shape in terms of curvature and twists, known as tortuosity. Tortuosity measurement and its automatic grading were discussed in various literature[28,29]. It should be considered that the tortuosity measurement is a parameter containing information on cardio and hypertension. Tortuosity changes its behaviors with respect to the change in the vessel due to hypertension and various vascular risk factors. However, it is still a challenge, and few literatures are available to find the association of ICP with tortuosity due to intracranial hypertension. The retinal tortuosity can be classified into parts as segmentation of tortuosity blood vessel followed by the tortuosity index measured value. The segmentation of the tortuosity is itself a challenging task; it generally affects the artery vein vessel without any clinical symptoms. The retinal tortuosity is usually curvature, and its behavior is non-uniform in determining it. For each curvature location, the pixel information is obtained from the centerline. The methods used include the measurement of retinal tortuosity using arc and chord method, Euclidean distance, Gabor angle at each segment in the curvature, circular Hough transforms and finding gradient on the curvature for different points. The tortuosity index (venous tortuosity and artery tortuosity) was measured using these various methods. Moss et al. [30] discussed the tortuosity associated with hypertension; further, elevated pressure can be a potential marker of ICP, which is related to elevated retinal venous pressures.

4 Results

The experiment results were carried out on the DRIVE database in this section. It consists of images containing a retinal fundus image and its segmented image manually performed by the experts. The segmentation of the retina fundus image in the proposed work is performed by learning the features while classifying the pixel. The dataset is trained and validated with the help of a deep learning architecture U-net for an epoch of 200. For optimizing the network SGD, ADAM and NADAM optimizer is used at a learning rate of 0.01 and 0.001. The learning rate is an important hyperparameter that controls the performance of the model. In training the model, a default learning rate of 0.01 has been considered initially, and then the performance of the model is tuned with different learning rates. At a learning rate of 0.001, the maximum accuracy is reached, while further increasing the learning rate, it results in a decrease in model performance. Table 3 and 4 depicts the performance of the network using various optimization algorithm for a batch size 4 and 8 at a different learning rate.

In Fig. 6, the accuracy of the artery and vein and its loss curve are shown for each epoch separately to validate the findings that the losses have been minimized. The individual accuracy of artery and vein is found to be 91.23 and 92.10, respectively. Further, the overall artery and vein segmentation accuracy is evaluated and illustrated in Fig. 7 with the respective loss curve. The results obtained optimal accuracy of 93.70 using the NADAM algorithm with a learning rate of 0.001 and batch size of 8. Further, the sensitivity and specificity were computed for the DRIVE database which found to be 92.35 and 93.41. This indicates that the proposed method can correctly predicts the artery and vein using the fundus image DRIVE database by hyper tuning the parameter.

Table 3. Performance of the network using various optimization algorithms (Batch Size = 4)

Optimizer	Parameter	Accuracy		
	Learning rate	Artery	Vein	Artery- Vein
SGD	Lr = 0.001	87.65	89.21	91.43
	Lr = 0.01	90.21	91.83	91.98
ADAM	Lr = 0.001	90.68	92.34	92.98
	Lr = 0.01	87.43	89.67	91.03
NADAM	Lr = 0.001	90.67	91.96	92.78
	Lr = 0.01	88.48	89.89	90.38

Table 4. Performance of the network using various optimization algorithms (Batch Size = 8)

Optimizer	Parameter	Accuracy		
	Learning rate	Artery	Vein	Artery- Vein
SGD	Lr = 0.001	88.31	90.10	89.43
	Lr = 0.01	88.64	91.47	91.89
ADAM	Lr = 0.001	90.78	91.76	92.43
	Lr = 0.01	89.89	88.20	92.67
NADAM	Lr = 0.001	**91.23**	**92.10**	**93.70**
	Lr = 0.01	89.35	90.78	92.71

Comparison with the Existing Methods:
The performance of our proposed approach on the DRIVE dataset is compared with the previous study's approaches. Table 5 illustrates the performance between the proposed method and the existing methods. The comparison is done on the artery-vein DRIVE

Table 5. Performance comparison of the artery vein on the DRIVE database

Methods	Accuracy
Dashtbozorg et al. [13]	87.4
Martinez-Perez et al. [14]	93.4
Estrada et al. [15]	93.5
Xu et al. [16]	92.3
Guo et al. [17]	91.9
Kang et al. [18]	90.8
Our Proposed	**93.7**

database, where artery and vein vessels are segmented using the deep learning approach. In evaluating the trained model, the testing accuracy is measured for the local dataset of 10 images which is not publicly available and obtained from the ophthalmologists. The proposed model achieved the testing accuracy of 92.97% for segmentation of the artery vein in the fundus image.

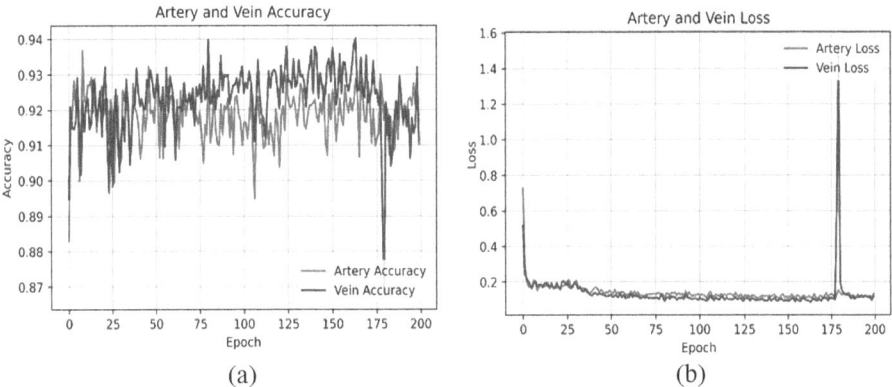

Fig. 6. Artery and Vein (a) accuracy curve, and (b) loss curve

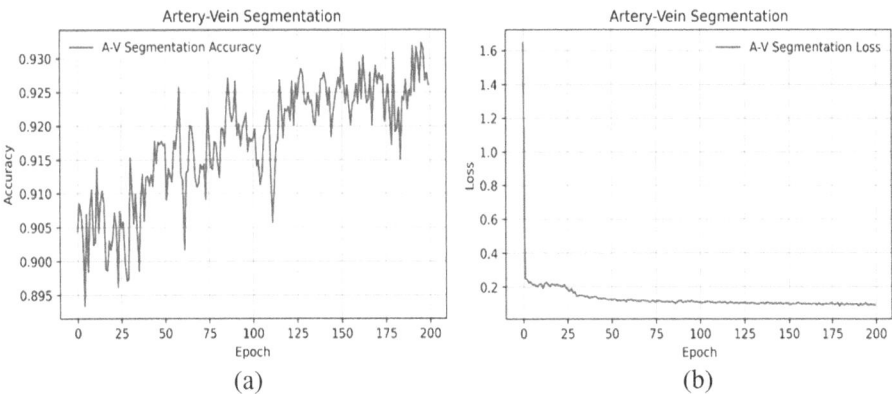

Fig. 7. Artery-Vein segmentation (a) accuracy curve and (b) loss curve

5 Discussion

The cause of high ICP can be fundamentally due to papilledema. The papilledema can be observed as obscuring vessels slowly by the swelling of axons, optic disc margin blurring, disc hyperemia accompanying capillaries enlargement, optic disc elevation, and narrowing of arteries in the nerve fiber layer. The invasive measurement has suggested that using lumbar puncture techniques for cerebrospinal fluid drainage lowers the

ICP and affects the retinal diameter proportionally. However, during the treatment of 6 months, there was a change in the retinal venule diameter and no changes in the arteriole diameter [31]. The automated measurement of retinal arteriole and venule diameter and its correlation need to be addressed to predict ICP. It is discussed in the literature that for the measurement of artery vein, the primary objective is to segment the vessels. The segmentation of the artery vein has particular challenges associated with its structure as:

1. It consists of different vessels with varying diameters, especially thin vessels. Thin vessel extraction and its measurement is a task.
2. The extraction of thin vessels may also be difficult sometimes if noise is present.
3. The localization of an artery and vein is confusing, and it may get misclassified sometimes while segmenting it.
4. Further, the artery-vein diameter measurement needs a deep learning automated module to predict the ICP for the trauma conditions.
5. The other challenges lie in differentiating the tortuosity concerning the artery vein and correlating these parameters with ICP, which is still unclear.

The optic CDR findings and their correlation with ICP findings is another challenge for trauma condition assessment;

1. In the CDR findings, the CDR in papilledema infected is 0.2 and 0.35 – 0.40 without papilledema [9].
2. Another study concludes that children with idiopathic intracranial hypertension have an absence of a cup, and the CDR is between 0.25 and 0.01.
3. It concludes that a limited study is currently present for correlating CDR in papilledema patients with ICP.
4. The study needs to be addressed; large sample size is needed.
5. The CDR findings with and without papilledema are still unclear for the ICP assessment in the trauma condition. The statistical analysis is needed for the correlation analysis.

This implies that future research will better understand various variable measurements using fundus imaging to assess ICP. The varying measurement techniques should also be precise when papilledema is not present in the retina.

6 Conclusion

This paper presented a segmentation method for the artery and vein in retinal fundus image using the deep learning architecture U-Net to assess the traumatic condition. The segmentation method of artery and vein can be further used for the diameter measurement of artery-vein diameter and tortuosity index. The cup to disc ratio (CDR) is another parameter which also correlated, and the various stages follow its measurement. The measurement of retinal arteriole and venule diameter, optic CDR, and tortuosity index can be marked for the analysis of the ICP using a retinal fundus image in future work. The measurement of the artery-vein diameter and its differentiation with tortuosity are needed while correlating ICP for the assessment. In another parameter, the measurement of optic CDR needed qualitative research for the screening where there should be clarity with the correlation of such patients who are suffering from papilledema.

References

1. Tang, A., et al.: Intracranial pressure monitors in patients with traumatic brain injury. J. Surg. Res. **194**(2), 565–570 (2015)
2. Singh, M., Kumar, B., Agrawal, D.: Good view frames from ultrasonography (USG) video containing ONS diameter using state-of-the-art deep learning architectures. Med. Biol. Eng. Comput. **60**, 3397–3417 (2022). https://doi.org/10.1007/s11517-022-02680-3
3. Bothwell, S.W., Janigro, D., Patabendige, A.: Cerebrospinal fluid dynamics and intracranial pressure elevation in neurological diseases. Fluids Barriers CNS **16**(1), 1–18 (2019)
4. Valova, G., Bogomyakova, O., Tulupov, A., Cherevko, A.: Influence of interaction of cerebral fluids on ventricular deformation: a mathematical approach. Plos one **17**(2), e0264395 (2022). 1371/jour-nal.pone.0264395
5. Doron, O., Zadka, Y., Barnea, O., Rosenthal, G.: Interactions of brain, blood, and CSF: a novel mathematical model of cerebral edema. Fluids Barriers CNS **18**(1), 1–14 (2021)
6. Mokri, B.: The monro-kellie hypothesis: applications in CSF volume depletion. Neurology **56**(12), 1746–1748 (2001)
7. Digre, K.B., Nakamoto, B.K., Warner, J.E., Langeberg, W.J., Baggaley, S.K., Katz, B.J.: A comparison of idiopathic intracranial hypertension with and without papilledema. Headache: J. Head Face Pain **49**(2), 185–193 (2009)
8. Kashif, F.M., Verghese, G.C., Novak, V., Czosnyka, M., Heldt, T.: Model-based non-invasive estimation of intracranial pressure from cerebral blood flow velocity and arterial pressure. Sci. Transl. Med. **4**(129), 129ra44–129ra44 (2012)
9. Hamill, E., Kim, J.D., Yalamanchili, S., Paranilam, J.M., Al Zubidi, N., Lee, A.G.: Cup-to-disc ratio in idiopathic intracranial hyper-tension without papilloedema. Neuro Ophthalmol. **38**(2), 69–73 (2014)
10. Saba, T., Akbar, S., Kolivand, H., Ali Bahaj, S.: Automatic detection of papilledema through fundus retinal images using deep learning. Micros. Res. Tech. **84**(12), 3066–3077 (2021)
11. Andersen, M.S., Pedersen, C.B., Poulsen, F.R.: A new novel method for assessing intracranial pressure using non-invasive fundus images: a pilot study. Sci. Rep. **10**(1), 1–7 (2020)
12. Ghate, D., et al.: The effects of acute intracranial pressure changes on the episcleral venous pressure, retinal vein diameter and intraocular pressure in a pig model. Curr. Eye Res. **46**(4), 524–531 (2021)
13. Dashtbozorg, B., Mendon¸ca, A.M., Campilho, A.: An automatic graph-based approach for artery/vein classification in retinal images. IEEE Trans. Image Process. **23**(3), 1073–1083 (2014)
14. Martinez-Perez, M.E., Hughes, A.D., Thom, S.A., Bharath, A.A., Parker, K.H.: Segmentation of blood vessels from red-free and fluorescein retinal images. Med. Image Anal. **11**(1), 47–61 (2007). https://doi.org/10.1016/j.media.2006.11.004
15. Estrada, R., Allingham, M.J., Mettu, P.S., Cousins, S.W., Tomasi, C., Farsiu, S.: Retinal artery-vein classification via topology estimation. IEEE Trans. Med. Imaging **34**(12), 2518–2534 (2015)
16. Xu, X., Ding, W., Abr'amoff, M.D., Cao, R.: An improved arteriovenous classification method for the early diagnostics of various diseases in retinal image. Comput. Methods Programs Biomed. **141**, 3–9 (2017), 119–126. Springer, Cham (2018). https://doi.org/10.1007/978-3-030-00934-2
17. Guo, Y., Budak, Ü., Vespa, L.J., Khorasani, E., Şengür, A.: A retinal vessel detection approach using convolution neural network with reinforcement sample learning strategy. Measurement **125**, 586–591 (2018)
18. Kang, H., Gao, Y., Guo, S., Xu, X., Li, T., Wang, K.: AVNet: a retinal artery/vein classification network with category-attention weighted fusion. Comput. Methods Programs Biomed. **195**, 105629 (2020). https://doi.org/10.1016/j.cmpb.2020.105629

19. Bailliart, O., Kedra, A.W., Bonnin, P., Savin, E., Martineaud, J.P.: Effects of bisoprolol on local vascular resistance. Eur. Heart J. Suppl M, 87–93. PMID: 2897303 (1987). https://doi.org/10.1093/eurheartj/8.suppl_m.87
20. Firsching, R., Müller, C., Pauli, S.-U., Voellger, B., Röhl, F.-W., Behrens-Baumann, W.: Non-invasive assessment of intracranial pressure with venous ophthalmodynamometry. J. Neurosurg. **115**(2), 371–374 (2011)
21. Wong, S.H., White, R.P.: The clinical validity of the spontaneous retinal venous pulsation. J. Neuro-Ophthalmol. **33**(1), 17–20 (2013)
22. D'Antona, L., et al.: Association of intracranial pressure and spontaneous retinal venous pulsation. JAMA Neurol. **76**(12), 1502–1505 (2019)
23. He, Y., et al.: Association between blood pressure and retinal arteriolar and venular diameters in Chinese early adolescent children, and whether the association has gender difference: a cross-sectional study. BMC Ophthalmol. **18**(1), 1–12 (2018)
24. Akbar, S., Akram, M.U., Sharif, M., Tariq, A., ullah Yasin, U.: Arteriovenous ratio and papilledema based hybrid decision support system for detection and grading of hypertensive retinopathy. Comput. Methods Programs Biomed. **154**, 123–141 (2018)
25. Geddie, B.E., Altiparmak, U.E., Eggenberger, E.R.: Cup-to-disc ratio in patients with idiopathic intracranial hypertension is smaller than that in normal subjects. J. Neuroophthalmol. **30**(3), 231–234 (2010)
26. Dai, S., Trimboli, C., Buncic, J.R.: The optic disc is minimal in children with idiopathic intracranial hypertension. J. Child Neurol. **28**(10), 1245–1249 (2013)
27. Horsburgh, J., Bativala, R., Burdon, M., Shah, P.: Early loss of optic cup with increased intracranial pressure. Neuro-Ophthalmol. **42**(5), 295–298 (2018)
28. Grisan, E., Foracchia, M., Ruggeri, A.: A novel method for the automatic grading of retinal vessel tortuosity. IEEE Trans. Med. Imaging **27**(3), 310–319 (2008)
29. Kalitzeos, A.A., Lip, G.Y., Heitmar, R.: Retinal vessel tortuosity measures and their applications. Exp. Eye Res. **106**, 40–46 (2013)
30. Moss, H.E., Cao, J., Wasi, M., Feldon, S.E., Shahidi, M.: Variability of retinal vessel tortuosity measurements using a semiautomated method applied to fundus images in subjects with papilledema. Transl. Vis. Sci. Technol. **10**(14), 32 (2021)
31. Moss, H.E., Hollar, R.A., Fischer, W.S., Feldon, S.E.: Retinal vessel diameter changes after 6 months of treatment in the idiopathic in-tracranial hypertension treatment trial. Br. J. Ophthalmol. **104**(10), 1430–1434 (2020)

A 1D-Convolutional Neural Network Framework with Multi-Modal Techniques for Sleep Staging System Using EEG and EOG Signals

Santosh Kumar Satapathy[1(✉)], Hari Kishan Kondaveeti[2], and Vaishvi R. Shah[1]

[1] Information and Communication Technology, Pandit Deendayal Energy University, Gandhinagar, Gujarat 382007, India
`Santosh.Satapathy@sot.pdpu.ac.in`
[2] School of Computer Science Engineering, VIT-AP University, Vijayawada, Andhra Pradesh 522237, India

Abstract. The objective is to develop a higher-performing automated sleep staging system by exploiting multi-modal polysomnography signal recordings . Three modalities of PSG signals, namely electroencephalogram (EEG) and electromyogram (EOG) were considered to obtain the optimal fusions of the PSG signals, where 63 features were extracted. These include frequency-based, time-based, statistical-based, entropy-based, and non-linear-based features. We adopted the ReliefF feature selection algorithms to find the suitable parts for each signal and superposition of PSG signals. Twelve top features were selected while correlated with the extracted feature sets' sleep stages. The selected features were fed into the one-dimensional convolutional neural network to validate the chosen segments and classify the sleep stages. This study's experiments were investigated by obtaining epoch-wise testing schemes. The proposed research was performed on the sleep-EDF(S-EDF) public dataset. In this work, we demonstrated that the proposed fusion strategy overestimates the common individual usage of PSG signals. The proposed experimental results reported an overall accuracy of 98.97%, 97.89%, 89.81%, 83.83%, and 83.72% for distinguishing between 'rapid eye movement stage (REM) vs. non-rapid eye movement stage (NREM),' 'deep sleep (NREM-N3 + NREM-N4) vs. light sleep (NREM-N1 + NREM-N2)', 'wake vs. sleep (NREM + REM),' and 'wake, deep sleep (NREM-N3 + NREM-N4)', 'light sleep (NREM-N1 + NREM-N2), and REM', 'wake, N1, N2, N3, and REM' respectively.

Keywords: CNN · EEG · EOG · Sleep Staging · Sleep Disorders · Deep learning

1 Introduction

On average, human beings spend one-third of their lives in sleep. As it occupies such a significant part of our lives, it is essential to understand sleep in as much depth as possible [1]. It can be defined as a state of active unconsciousness in which the brain is in a relatively relaxed state and reacts to various internal stimuli because of a reduction in sensory perception [2]. An 8-h sleep consists of 4–5 cycles; each cycle lasting approximately 90 min. These cycles contain various sleep stages which can mainly be divided into Wakefulness(W), NREM (Non-Rapid Eye Movement), and REM (Rapid Eye Movement), where REM sleep increases as the night progresses. NREM can further be divided into light sleep(N1), deeper light sleep(N2), and slow wave sleep (N3) [3]. Sleep plays several fundamental biological functions in our bodies, allowing for maintenance, repair, and building of the body and so, is important in maintaining and improving physical and mental health. Despite this, many people get less than the recommended amount of sleep or suffer from sleeping disorders. By addressing potential underlying sleep disorders such as insomnia and sleep apnea as well as constant attention to sleep hygiene and lifestyle modification, one can substantially improve health [4]. Due to these reasons, a systematic classification and analysis becomes essential.

Generally, sleep stages cannot be determined just by looking at an EEG signal; a structured process is necessary which is exactly what sleep staging aims to do. It is the process of classifying various sleep stages which helps to detect the quality of sleep [5]. For this entire process, all-night polysomnographic (PSG) recordings remain the most accurate source of data even today. The PSG recordings include electroencephalograms (EEGs) which are used as a tool to assess brain activity to identify the deep phase of sedation, electrooculograms (EOGs) which are essential for detecting REM sleep as they track eye movements and electromyograms (EMGs) which monitors heart rates. These are usually acquired from patients for a thorough analysis [3, 6]. Over the years, alternate methods have been suggested for the sleep staging process. These alternatives include automatic sleep staging using cardiorespiratory signals as well as sleep staging based on a convolutional neural network (CNN). Although these methods aim to provide a clearer feature extraction, the high temporal resolution and established reliability that EEG has to offer makes it the most widely used dataset for this process [7, 8]. Moreover, with recent advances in technologies such as artificial intelligence, high-accuracy classification systems are available based on varied machine learning and deep learning approaches for larger PSG dataset analysis eradicating the existing problems and making EEGs widely popular for analysis purposes.

2 Related Work

The authors present an innovative technique utilizing EEG data to detect sleep-related issues. The method involves three key phases: feature extraction, classification, and data preparation. Integrating an Ensemble Machine Learning Classifier alongside Hybrid Deep Learning yields a significant enhancement in classification accuracy, achieving 96.78%, and sensitivity, reaching 89.06% [3].

In a related study, the authors propose an advanced approach employing EEG data for sleep problem identification. The methodology encompasses three primary stages: feature extraction, classification, and data preparation. Through the incorporation of an Ensemble Machine Learning Classifier combined with Hybrid Deep Learning, there is a noteworthy improvement in classification accuracy, attaining 96.78%, and sensitivity, reaching 89.06% [4].

Additionally, the authors design a Convolutional Neural Network (CNN) architecture for predicting sleep quality. The CNN architecture comprises the Fully Linked Layer, Pooling Layer, and Convolutional Layer. The CNN model is trained on a series of sensor data readings obtained through wearable technology, reflecting user movement, heart rate, and breathing rate measurements. The model achieves high accuracy, with results of 93% on the PSD dataset and 95% on the SHHRS dataset [5].

The authors have introduced a deep learning model named OxiNet, based on single-channel oximetry, for detecting obstructive sleep apnea (OSA). OxiNet, a Convolutional Neural Network (CNN) model, predicts the apnea-hypopnea index (AHI) – a severity measure for OSA derived from apnea and hypopnea occurrences per sleep hour. Utilizing a single-channel oximetry signal, a time series of blood oxygen saturation (SpO2), OxiNet achieves a sensitivity of 78% and an accuracy of 97% [6].

Another research effort presents a deep learning system designed to automatically stage sleep using instantaneous heart rate (IHR) data. The system employs a CNN architecture to learn temporal patterns in IHR data corresponding to different sleep phases. Trained on a dataset containing IHR information and sleep phases from over 10,000 sleep study nights, the CNN receives IHR values sampled at 1 Hz and provides sleep stage predictions for each 30-s IHR data sequence. The CNN algorithm achieves an overall accuracy of 77% [7].

Furthermore, the study proposes SleepInceptionNet, a CNN-based model, the model includes a preprocessing layer for normalizing and filtering input data, multiple convolutional layers for feature extraction, pooling layers to reduce data dimensionality, and fully connected layers for categorizing extracted features into sleep stages. The polysomnography data incorporates EEG signals from various channels, along with other physiological signals like EOG (eye movements) and EMG (muscle activity). The model achieves a Cohen's kappa value of 0.705, and it is noted that an Artificial Neural Network (ANN) architecture can be employed as an alternative to CNN [8].

In [9], the author introduces a novel method for sleep stage classification using a joint approach of quaternion-valued singular spectrum analysis (QSSA) and ensemble empirical mode decomposition (EEMD). Computer simulations demonstrate the effectiveness of QSSA in noise suppression, and the bagging classifier, utilizing statistical features from both QSSA components and intrinsic mode functions (IMFs), achieves accurate sleep stage classification.

In [10], the study explores the sleep stage classification using 232 features derived from these PSG signals, encompassing statistical, frequency, time-frequency, fractal, entropy, and nonlinear characteristics. The random forest classifier achieves an optimal accuracy of 86.24%.

In [11], the focus is on scoring sleeping EEG signals to assess the impact of feature reduction techniques on increasing pressure on features. The study also explores the advantages of increasing the number of input signals to allow the network to extract better features.

In [12], the author used SVM techniques and the average accuracy achieved was 96.74% based on AASM standards and 96% based on R&K standards.

In [13], the author directly applies the raw EEG signal to a deep convolutional neural network without feature extraction/selection. The proposed network architecture achieves accuracy above 90% for classifying two up to six classes. The Kappa Cohen's coefficients indicate significant improvements compared to existing methods, ranging from 0.86 to 0.98.

To tackle the challenges outlined above, we present a model for signal fusion based on multi-modality, employing deep learning techniques. The primary contributions of our research are as follows:

- We introduce a multi-modality signal fusion approach to analyze and categorize sleep stage behaviors utilizing deep learning methods. This involves the application of 1D-CNN to automatically discern changes in the characteristics of sleep stages and capture significant waveform features present in both EEG and EOG signals.
- Our methodology adopts an end-to-end pipeline, wherein features are directly extracted from the raw single-channel EEG and EOG signals, eliminating the need for pre-processing methods in sleep staging.
- The proposed model yields promising results when tested on the Sleep-EDF dataset. Comparative assessments are conducted against recent studies utilizing the same single-channel EEG and EOG signals, validating the superior performance of our approach.

3 Materials and Methods

This section delineates the dataset description, pre-processing, and proposed 1D-CNN model followed by an overview of feature collection, the GA methodology, and the NN framework. Figure 1 offers a schematic representation of the proposed methodology.

3.1 Datasets

The sleep cassette dataset used for this research is sourced from the Sleep Physionet Dataset which is a publicly accessible database. It contains 153 files obtained from a 1987–1991 study of age effects on sleep in healthy Caucasians aged 25–101, without any sleep-related medication. The dataset consists of two types of files. The first type of files are PSG files which are whole-night polysomnographic recordings comprising EEG, EOG, and EMG readings along with an event marker (a time-stamped label). EEG (electroencephalogram) records the brain activity, EOG (electrooculogram) records the eye movements and EMG (electromyogram) records the muscle activity. These PSG files often contain oro-nasal respiration and rectal body temperature as well. For this particular study, only the EEG readings were crucial so the other measurements have been excluded during pre-processing. The second type of files are hypnogram files which contain annotations of the sleep patterns that correspond to the PSGs. These files, which are manually scored by well-trained technicians, consist of sleep stages W, REM, N1, N2, N3, and N4. The files are named in the form SC4482F0-PSG.edf where SC stands for sleep cassette. Each of the EEG signals is sampled at 100 Hz [15].

3.2 Preprocessing

Biomedical signals are captured from subjects using various electrodes placed on the skull. These raw signals may exhibit diverse magnitudes and are susceptible to

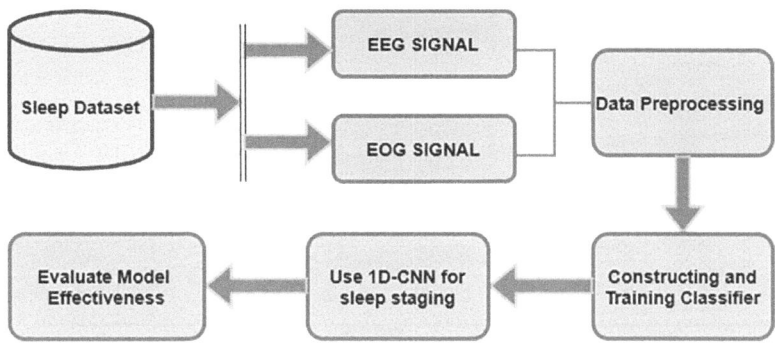

Fig. 1. Overview of the proposed sleep staging architecture

sensor non-linearity, noise, and various artifacts such as muscle twitching and motion, as well as eye blinks. In this study, classical methods are employed for scaling and normalization. This involves transforming the signals into normalized samples, with each signal having a mean (μ) and standard deviation (σ). To further enhance signal quality, artifacts are removed using a 10th-order Butterworth bandpass filter [16].

3.3 One-Dimensional Convolutional Neural Networks (1D-CNN)

The CNN model typically consists of multiple convolutional layers, a max-pooling layer, and one or more fully connected layers, and concludes with a softmax activation function determining output class probabilities. In this model, information transforms from one layer to the next. The initial layers capture low-level features, gradually progressing to deeper layers where more intricate information is extracted. Figure 2 illustrates the typical structure of a CNN model. Figure 3 illustrates the proposed 1D-CNN architecture.

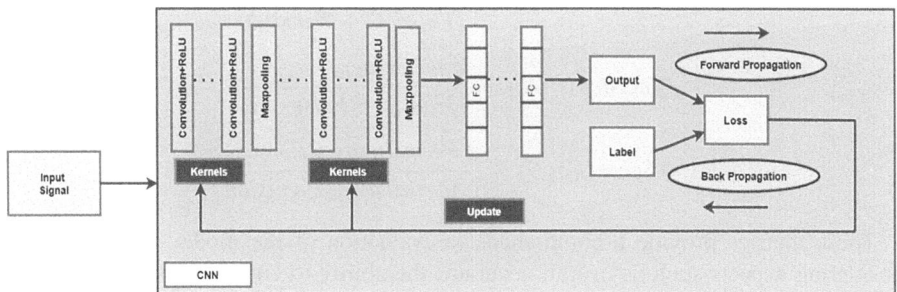

Fig. 2. Compositions of One-dimensional convolutional neural network

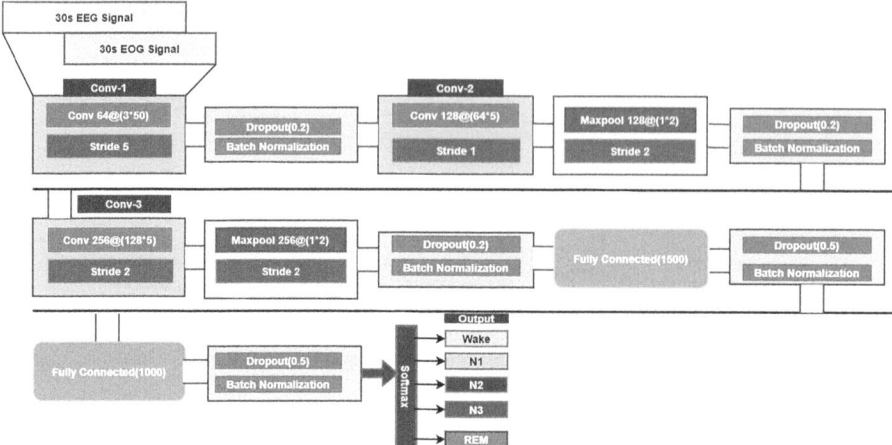

Fig. 3. The architecture of the proposed 1D-CNN model

3.4 Performance Assessment

To analyze the performance of the proposed model. We have used various metrics and their mathematical formulations for these metrics, denoted by Eqs. (1) through (5), are as follows:

$$Accuracy(Accu) = \frac{(True_{pos} + True_{neg})}{True_{pos} + True_{neg} + False_{pos} + False_{neg}} \quad (1)$$

$$Specificity(Spec) = \frac{True_{neg}}{(True_{neg} + False_{pos})} \quad (2)$$

$$Sensitivity(Sens) = \frac{True_{pos}}{(False_{neg} + True_{pos})} \quad (3)$$

$$Precision(Prec) = \frac{True_{pos}}{(True_{pos} + False_{pos})} \quad (4)$$

$$F1 - Score(F1\_S) = \frac{2 * Sensitivity * Precision}{Sensitivity + Precision} \quad (5)$$

These metrics provide a comprehensive evaluation of the model's performance, considering aspects such as overall accuracy, the ability to correctly identify positive instances (sensitivity), the ability to correctly identify negative instances (specificity), precision in positive predictions, and a balanced measure (F1-Score) that considers both precision and sensitivity. The adoption of these metrics facilitates a thorough analysis of the model's effectiveness.

4 Experimental Results

The experimentation on multi-class and binary sleep stages classification involved the utilization of the 1D-CNN model. Five distinct experiment cases were considered: (i) Wake vs. N1 vs. N2 vs. N3 vs. REM, (ii) Wake vs. Light Sleep (LS) vs. Deep Sleep (DS) vs. REM, (iii) REM vs. NREM, and (iv) Wake vs. Sleep. In each case, the proposed research work's performance was compared with state-of-the-art works in these specific experiments to evaluate its effectiveness and competitiveness.

The proposed model's ability to discriminate between different sleep stages in these experiments was analyzed and benchmarked against existing research, providing insights into its comparative performance in each specific classification task. This comprehensive evaluation aimed to highlight the strengths and contributions of the proposed approach in advancing the state of the art in sleep stage classification using the 1D-CNN model.

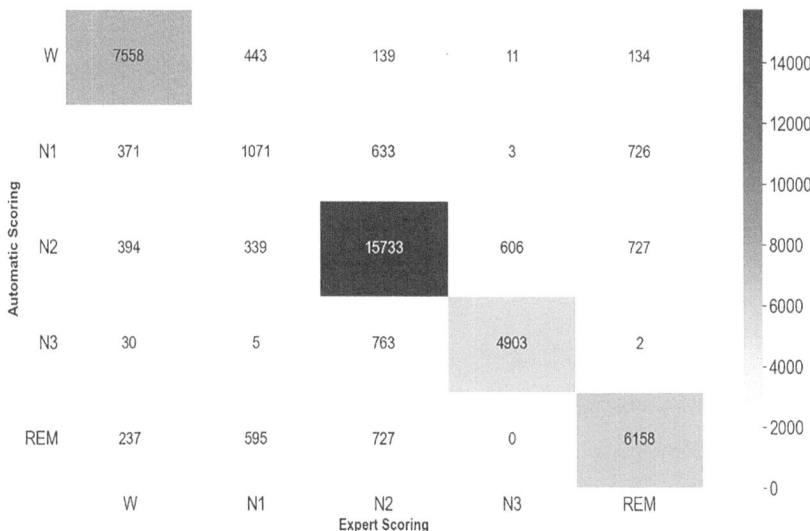

Fig. 4. Generated confusion matrix from the proposed model for a five-class classification problem using EEG + EOG signals

Figure 4 illustrates the confusion matrix obtained for five-class classification problems. Similarly, Figs. 5, 6, 7 and 8 depict the confusion matrices for four-class (Wake vs. Light Sleep vs. Deep Sleep vs. REM), two-class (Non-REM vs. REM), two-class (Light Sleep vs. Deep Sleep), and two-class (Wake vs. Sleep), respectively. The model achieved commendable classification accuracy rates, specifically 98.79% for two-class (Non-REM vs. REM), 91.07% for two-class (Light Sleep vs. Deep Sleep), and 89.81% for two-class (Wake vs. Non-REM + REM). For the more challenging five-class and four-class classification problems, the model reported accuracies of 83.72% and 83.83%, respectively. Figure 9 illustrates achieved accuracies for multi-class and binary-class sleep stage classification problems. Similarly, Fig. 10 presents a summary of the performance metric for each sleep stage. To assess the proposed system's effectiveness, a

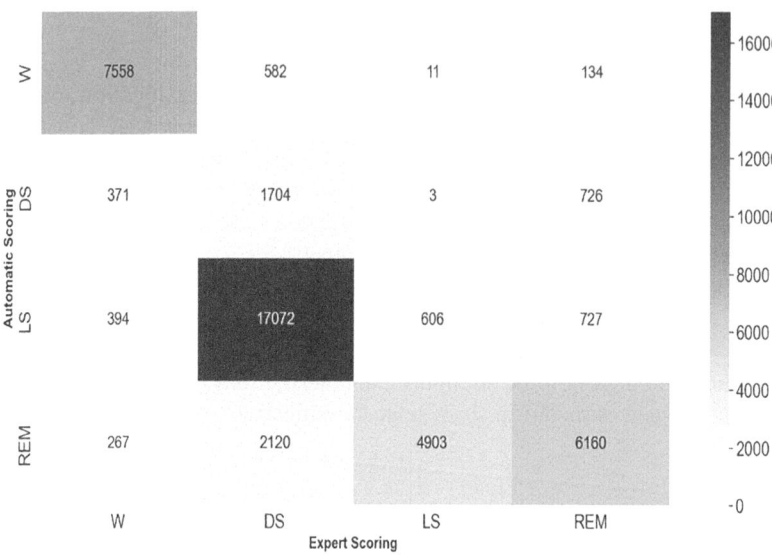

Fig. 5. Obtained confusion matrix from the proposed model for a four-class classification problem using EEG + EOG signals

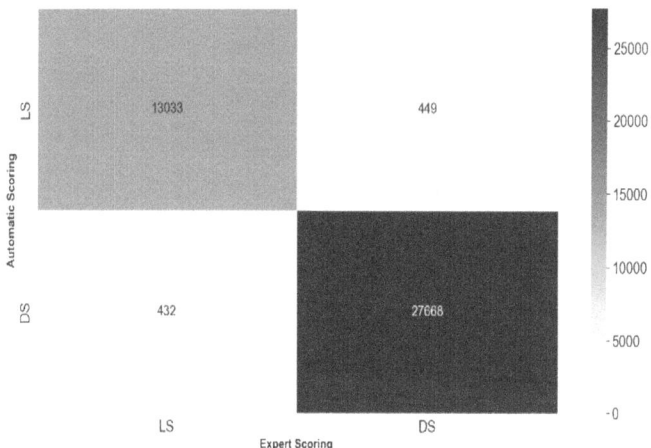

Fig. 6. The confusion matrix of two-class (LS vs DS) sleep staging using EEG + EOG signals

comparison with state-of-the-art works was conducted. Figure 11 illustrates the comparisons of the results. The proposed model demonstrates competitive performance, emphasizing its efficacy in sleep stage classification.

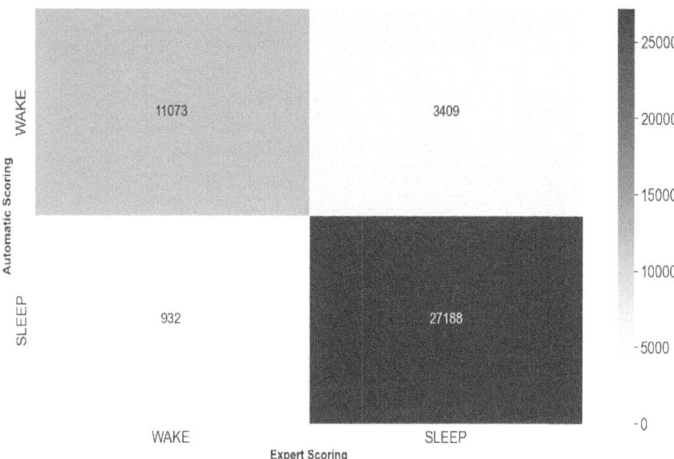

Fig. 7. The confusion matrix of two-class (Wake vs. Sleep) sleep staging with the 1D-CNN model using EEG + EOG signals

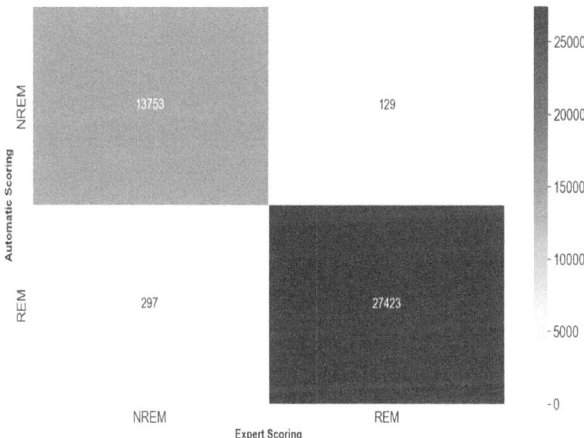

Fig. 8. The confusion matrix of two-class (NREM vs. REM) sleep staging using EEG + EOG signals

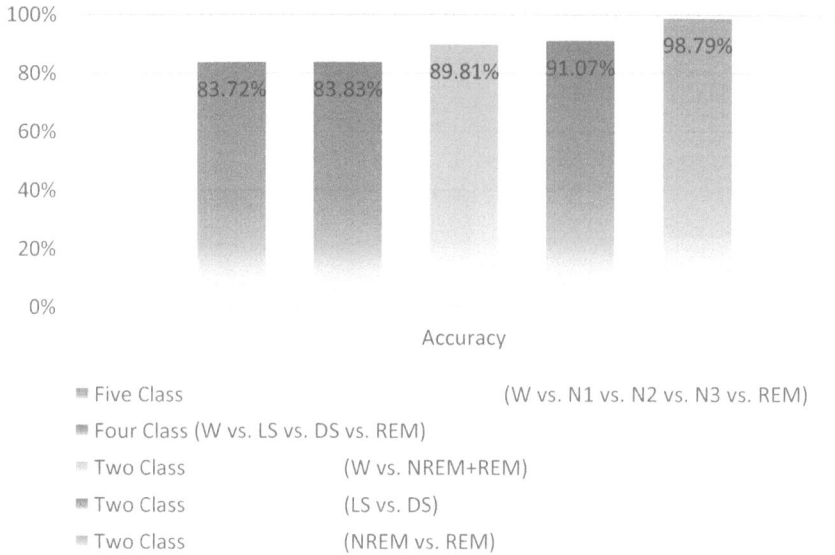

Fig. 9. Accuracies for five-class, four-class, and two-class sleep stages classification problems using the S-EDF database with EEG + EOG signals

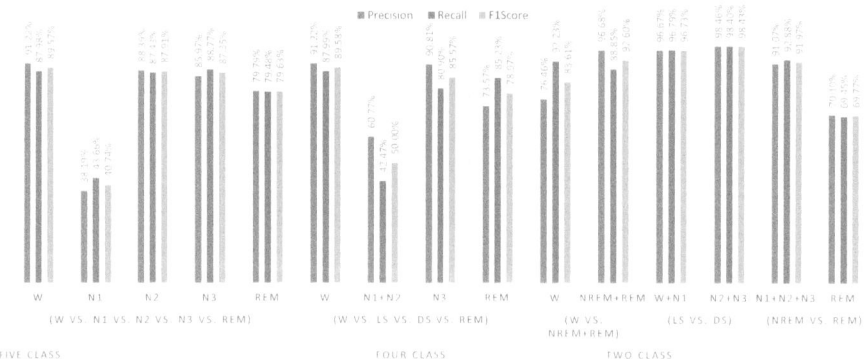

Fig. 10. Performance metrics of proposed sleep staging method on Sleep-EDF database using EEG + EOG signals

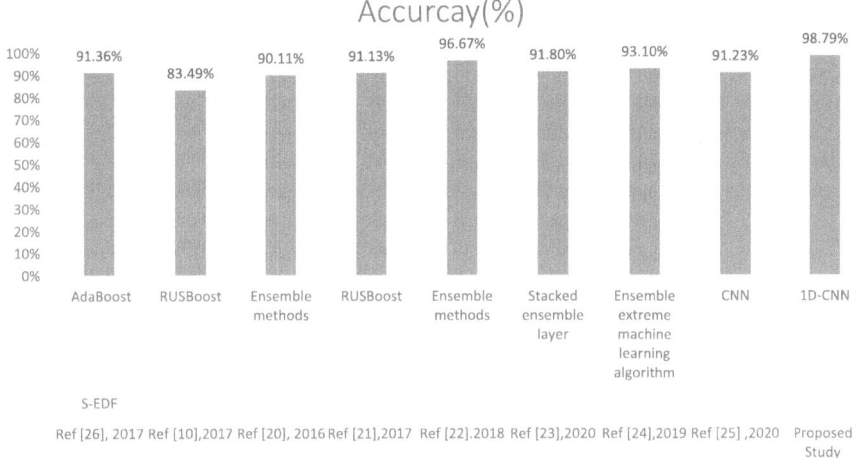

Fig. 11. Performance comparisons between proposed model and different state-of-the-art works

5 Conclusion

Precise and efficient sleep staging holds significant importance in the analysis and detection of sleep irregularities. In this research work a sleep staging system to enhance accuracy and robustness in automatic sleep stage classification, addressing both multi-class and two-class sleep state classification issues. The proposed system utilizes a multi-modal approach for signal fusion, incorporating polysomnography signals. The model's performance was evaluated on the widely accepted S-EDF dataset, comprising sleep recordings from subjects with various sleep-related disorders and healthy controls, each of 30-s duration. The experiments were conducted on an epoch-wise basis. Results from the experiments indicate the superiority of the proposed methodology employing multi-modal signal fusions over alternative machine learning classification models. Future work aims to expand the proposed approach by integrating different physiological signals, facilitating the detection of multiple types of simulated sleep disorders.

References

1. Li, Y., Peng, C., Zhang, Y., Zhang, Y., Lo, B.: Adversarial learning for semi-supervised pediatric sleep staging with single-EEG channel. Method **204**, 84–91 (2022). ISSN 1046-2023. https://doi.org/10.1016/j.ymeth.2022.03.013
2. Satapathy, S.K., Loganathan, D.: Automated classification of sleep stages using single-channel EEG: a machine learning-based method. Int. J. Inform. Retri. Res. (IJIRR), **12**(2), 1–19 (2022). https://doi.org/10.4018/IJIRR.299941
3. Saran, R., Kumar, A., Srivastava, H.B.: Real-Time Parallel Computing De-sign for Implementation of Point/Small Target Detection Algorithm in Visible/Infra-Red Video. In: 2018 Fifth International Conference on Parallel, Distributed and Grid Computing (PDGC), pp. 300–305 (2018). https://doi.org/10.1109/PDGC.2018.8745829

4. Singh, V., Asari, V.K., Rajasekaran, R.: A deep neural network for early detection and prediction of chronic kidney disease. Diagnostics **12**(1), 116 (2022). https://doi.org/10.3390/diagnostics12010116
5. Rastogi, P., Khanna, K., Singh, V.: Gland segmentation in colorectal cancer histopathological images using U-net inspired convolutional network. Neural Comput. Appl. **34**, 5383–5395 (2022). https://doi.org/10.1007/s00521-021-06687-z
6. Satapathy, S., Loganathan, D., Kondaveeti, H.K. et al.: Performance analysis of machine learning algorithms on automated sleep staging feature sets. CAAI Trans. Intell. Technol. **6**(2), 155–174 (2021). https://doi.org/10.1049/cit2.12042
7. Widasari, E.R., Tanno, K., Tamura, H.: Automatic sleep disorders classification using ensemble of bagged tree based on sleep quality features. Electronics **9**(3), 512 (2020). https://doi.org/10.3390/electronics9030512
8. Satapathy, S.K., Loganathan, D.: Automated classification of multi-class sleep stages classification using polysomnography signals: a nine-layer 1D-convolution neural network approach. Multimed. Tools Appl. (2022). https://doi.org/10.1007/s1042022-13195-2
9. Huang, Z., Wing-Kuen Ling, B.: Sleeping stage classification based on joint quaternion valued singular spectrum analysis and ensemble empirical mode decomposition. Biomed. Sig. Process. Control **71**, Part A, 103086 (2022). ISSN 1746-8094. https://doi.org/10.1016/j.bspc.2021.103086
10. Yan, R., et al.: Multi-modality of polysomnography signals' fusion for automatic sleep scoring. Biomed. Sig. Process. Control **49**, 14–23 (2019). ISSN 1746-8094. https://doi.org/10.1016/j.bspc.2018.10.001
11. Fernandez-Blanco, E., Rivero, D., Pazos, A.: EEG signal processing with separable convolutional neural network for automatic scoring of sleeping stage, Neurocomputing **410**, 220–228 (2020). ISSN 0925-2312. https://doi.org/10.1016/j.neucom.2020.05.085
12. Diykh, M., Li, Y., Abdulla, S.: EEG sleep stages identification based on weighted undirected complex networks. Comput. Methods Programs Biomed. **184**, 105116 (2020). ISSN 0169-2607. https://doi.org/10.1016/j.cmpb.2019.105116
13. Wang, H., Guo, H., Zhang, K., Gao, L., Zheng, J.: Automatic sleep staging method of EEG signal based on transfer learning and fusion network. Neurocomputing **488**, 183–193 (2022). ISSN 0925-2312. https://doi.org/10.1016/j.neucom.2022.02.049
14. Zhang, C., Liu, S., Han, F., Nie, Z., Lo, B., Zhang, Y.: Hybrid manifold-deep convolutional neural network for sleep staging. Methods **202**, 164–172 (2022). ISSN 1046-2023. https://doi.org/10.1016/j.ymeth.2021.02.014
15. Li, Y., Peng, C., Zhang, Y., Zhang, Y., Lo, B.: Adversarial learning for semi-supervised pediatric sleep staging with the single-EEG channel. Methods **204**, 84–91 (2022). ISSN 1046-2023. https://doi.org/10.1016/j.ymeth.2022.03.013
16. Li, F., et al.: End-to-end sleep staging using convolutional neural network in raw single-channel EEG. Biomed. Sig. Process. Control **63**, 102203 (2021). ISSN 1746-8094. https://doi.org/10.1016/j.bspc.2020.102203
17. Jain, R., Ganesan, R.A.: Reliable sleep staging of unseen subjects with fusion of multiple EEG features and RUSBoost. Biomed. Sig. Process. Control **70**, 103061 (2021). ISSN 1746-8094. https://doi.org/10.1016/j.bspc.2021.103061
18. Satapathy, S.K., Loganathan, D.: Prognosis of automated sleep staging based on two-layer ensemble learning stacking model using single-channel EEG signal. Soft. Comput. **25**, 15445–15462 (2021). https://doi.org/10.1007/s00500-021-06218-x
19. Zhu, G., Li, Y., Wen, P.: Analysis and classification of sleep stages based on difference visibility graphs from a single-channel EEG signal. IEEE J. Biomed. Health Inform. **18**(6), 1813–1821, November 2014. https://doi.org/10.1109/JBHI.2014.2303991
20. Hassan, A.R., Bhuiyan, M.I.H.: Automatic sleep scoring using statistical features in the EMD domain and ensemble methods. Biocybern. Biomed. Eng. **36**(1), 248–255 (2016)

21. Rahman, M.M., Bhuiyan, M.I.H., Hassan, A.R.: Sleep stage classification using single-channel EOG. Comput. Biol. Med. **102**, 211–220, 1 Nov 2018. https://doi.org/10.1016/j.compbiomed.2018.08.022
22. Sharma, M., Goyal, D., Achuth, P.: Acharya, UR (2018) An accurate sleep stage classification system using a new class of optimally time-frequency localized three-band wavelet filter bank. Comput. Biol. Med. **98**, 58–75 (2018)
23. Zhou, J., et al.: Automatic sleep stage classification with single channel EEG signal based on two-layer stacked ensemble model. IEEE Access 1 (2020). https://doi.org/10.1109/access.2020.2982434
24. Abdulla, S., Diykh, M., Laft, R.L., Saleh, K., Deo, R.C.: Sleep EEG signal analysis based on correlation graph similarity coupled with an ensemble extreme machine learning algorithm. Expert Syst. Appl. (2019). https://doi.org/10.1016/j.eswa.2019.07.007
25. Zhou, Y., Zhao, D.: Application of convolutional neural network-based biosensor and electroencephalogram signal in sleep staging. J. Amb. Intell. Hum. Comput. (2021). https://doi.org/10.1007/s12652-021-03076-1
26. Hassan, A.R., Bhuiyan, M.I.H.: An automated method for sleep staging from EEG signals using normal inverse Gaussian parameters and adaptive boosting. Neurocomputing **204**, 76–87 (2017). ISSN 0925-2312 https://doi.org/10.1016/j.neucom.2016.09.011

Review on Mental Healthcare System Using Data Analytics and IoT

Mrinmoy Kayal[✉], Mohinikanta Sahoo, and Jayadeep Pati

Department of Computer Science and Engineering, Indian Institute of Information Technology Ranchi, Ranchi, Jharkhand 834010, India
mrinmoy02.rs21@iiitranchi.ac.in

Abstract. Today many people are suffering from mental illness in the world. Mental illnesses are health conditions involving changes in emotion, thinking or behavior and it associates with distress and functional problems in social, family activities. The aim of this paper shows how to examine about the mental illness using big data analytics. This review paper also presents a comparative analysis of different data analytics algorithms for mental healthcare. We have given a details description about five types of mental illness such as anxiety, depression, mood, bipolar, personality disorders and their effect of mental health on patient's natures and characteristics such as Suicide and drug addiction. Artificial intelligence and machine learning are used for prediction about the mental patient such as their behavior. IoT is also used for smart devices like smart watches and innovative bands to measure the mental healthcare system.

Keywords: Big data · AI · Machine learning · IoT · mental healthcare system

1 Introduction

"Big data" has most important things all over the world. Today, big data helps the medical research and public health strategies. The scientists have been providing the health care information to the patients by analyzing the big data analytics. There are several data sources such as patient clinical records, hospital records, medical exam results in the mental health care and these are valuable information store for predictive analysis. There are lots of applications of IoT in mental healthcare such as monitoring, diagnosis and treatment of the patients. IoT is a process of communication in which has one network device shares or exchanges the information to another network device in De la Torre Díez et al. [27].

In mental healthcare system, data is an information that is coming from different types of the sources, one is providers (patient's details and prescription) and another is non providers (searching engine) in khattak et al. [1]. Big data has been interpreted different modes and predict the future data which gets the final result. There are many researchers working on AI and big data analytics to solve the future data and analysis of big raw data and extract helpful data from it. Many researchers have been developed the AI algorithm and variety of wearable sensors which are used to predict the patient disease. Today increasing the health care technique, lots of mobile apps and smart devices such as wearable sensor devices are used in mobile mental healthcare systems. Many researchers have been working on AI and ML algorithms to predict the future data and to analyze the raw data. This raw data in healthcare is to manage very difficult with traditional database management tools because it is a big data which is in terabytes and petabytes.

In this paper, we analyze three sections about the mental health care using big data. The first section, we explain the literature review related to mental healthcare.. The second section, explains about different types mental disorders and it's effects. At the last section, describes on the discussion about mental disorder or illness using data science.

2 Literature Review

We have been studied and analyzed 28 papers. Bauer et al. [2] had been presented survey paper of bipolar disorder in which 1222 patients from 17 countries were entered and detect the bipolar disorder about older and younger adults. 12 different languages were translated in this survey. The datasets were collected from US Research University that analyzed text messages and phone calls to check the personality of the user in De Monyjoye [3]. Bleidorn [4] presented about personality assessment using machine learning. Digital healthcare innovation was presented in the paper Hill et al. [5]. In Monteith et al. [7], the survey analyzed about big data to provide the psychiatry data. Yang et al. [10], an IoT structured long-term wearable social sensing about mental patients were explained here that how to monitor the patients and how to sense the environment using wearable devices. Using automated decision making algorithm for disease, the collected data were analyzed in Monteith and Glenn [11]. These data were searching for hit disease website, email and distributed information on the social media. Goyal [12] presented about the twitter data which were filtered regarding food crisis and public opinion. Kumar and Bala [13] proposed about mental health data using MongoDB. Turner et al. [16], analyzed about healthcare using big data in automated decision making. I.C.Passions et al. [17], analyzed about the mental healthcare using machine learning and big data. A system literature review presents in the following table 1 which shows the appearance of big data chronologically in different types mental disorders.

3 Mental Disorder, Types and Effects

There are five types of mental disorders describe in literature which are presented as follows:

Anxiety Disorder. Anxiety is a normal emotion in which many people worry about things such as health, money and family problems. Anxiety disorders are different types of mental health condition which makes difficult life through the whole day.

If anyone has an anxiety disorder, he or she may respond to fear or dread situations in a certain manner and have experience of physical signs of anxiety which shows as pounding

Table 1. Study on Different types mental disorders.

Reference no	Reviewed topic	Methodology	No of reviewed paper	Topic analysis
3	Personality assessment	Big data, CDR	31	Analyzing text messages and phone calls
5	Mental disorder	Mental health, e-therapies CBT Platform	33	Developing smart phone and analysis e-therapies
22	Personality disorder	Dark side, big five, facet analysis, dependence and dutifulness	34	Analysis all the personality disorders
4	Personality assessment	Machine learning, big data	65	Develop the assessment tools to Predict the human behavior using ML
9	Mental wellbeing	Wearable device using smart devices	66	Long term monitoring experiment with wellbeing questionnaires
2	Bipolar disorder	Documentary survey	68	Analysis 47% of older adults and 87% of younger adults having bipolar disorder
8	Big brain data	Machine learning, big data	77	Analyze maximizing medical knowledge, security and the confidentiality of brain data

heart and sweating. There are several types of anxiety disorder such as generalized, panic, obsessive-compulsive, post-traumatic stress and social anxiety disorder P.Dhaka [14].

Depression Disorder. Depression is a common mental health condition in which it is major or clinical condition where feeling sad or hopeless. Depression can also cause difficulty with thinking, eating, memory and sleeping. Without treatment of depression, it can get very bad and last longer. In most cases, it can happen to self harm or death.

Bipolar Disorder. Bipolar disorder is also type of mental disorder that causes tremendous mood swings that include high emotional such as mania or hypomania and low emotion such as depression. In the table, Bauer et al.[2] surveying the bipolar disorder about adults, 187 older adults and 1021 younger adults data were collected from 17 countries. In survey, there were 39 questions and provided 20 min to complete the answer. We surveyed that younger adults were more addicted than the older adults.

Mood Disorder. Mood disordered is the one type mental disorder that the primarily effects of emotional state. It can cause changes the behavior such as persistent, intense sadness, anger. The mood disorder afflicts 9.4 millons American like mania and bipolar disorder P.Dhaka [14].

Personality Disorder. Personality disorder is also type mental disorder that exists the dutifulness in which the patients are much more stressed about the disease. It is a group of mental illness which involves long term thoughts and behavior that are unhealthy. Today, this type of disorder is not decreased, it's increasing day by day Furnham [22].

Effect of Mental Disorder

Mental disorder is a mental health condition that feelings danger, fear, helplessness and sadness of the people. Some issues of the mental disorder such as suicide, opioid and drug abuse as follows.

 i. **Suicide**: Suicide is a problem of the situation that self directed potentially injurious behavior with intent to die as a result behavior. Every minute a people dies from the suicide according to the researches opinion. Mental disorder and suicide are scattered all over the world and 90% of the people died by suicide according to khattak[1]. We analyze machine learning and big data can be used to predict suicides of depressed person. There are many tools in which can be used such as python anaconda, Jupiter notebook, Numpy, Pandas, Matplotlib and also analyzed the correlations using pearson's.
 ii. **Opioid**: Opioid is a type drugs and a substance which used to treat moderate to severe pain. Upperlimit of An opioid, can reverse the drug naloxone when give right away.
 iii. **Drugs abuse**: Many people have been used to take drugs but most of them are addicted the drugs at higher limit for feeling relaxed, it causes a problem. Adderall divinorum, snus, bath salts are all the drugs. Opioid is a type of drugs which used the illegitimate drug heroin. Hasan et al. [20] using random forest, decision tree, logistic regression and gradient boosting to predict about the opioid in mental disordered. According to Granka [24], information searches about the behavior measures of individual's interest in the issue.

4 Discussion About How Does Big Data Help to Predict Mental Disorder:

Now a days there are lots of medical mobile devices which have been used to set up in patient's body networks. These devices have been received and transmit the records of medical data for patient's evaluation by the doctors. There are lots of techniques to develop the mental healthcare data processing on cellular gadgets.

Table 2. Study of effect of mental disorder

Reference no	Topic	Effect	Methodology	Result
18	Personality disorder	Suicide	ML algorithm	Predict the risk of suicide
19	Psychological or personality disorder	Antidepressant usage	Cluster analysis	Identify the correlation between antidepressant and deprivation
20	Mental Pain of patient	Opioid	Logistic regression Random forest Gradient boosting	Suppressing the increasing rate of opioid addiction using ML
21	Psychological or personality disorder	Drug abuse	Google search history, monitoring the future data	Provide real time data to predict abuse and quickly respond
28	Borderline Personality Disorder	Suicide, Fear of abandonment, inappropriate anger	BPD(Borderline Personality Disorder) Neural Network	Etiological hypothesis of BPD

Effect of mental disorder and their solution using big data of Table 2.

There are three things such as AI, big data and social media to predict about the mental disorder. Big data is group of data sets in which are abundant and intricate in character. Wearable tracking devices and electronic records have been providing the data to store huge amount of data. Smart mobile Apps can be predicted different types healthcare problems such as mental, heart attack, emotion detection and calculate ECG. In Dimitrov [6], the combination of IOT and AI to create the healthcare apps so that easily

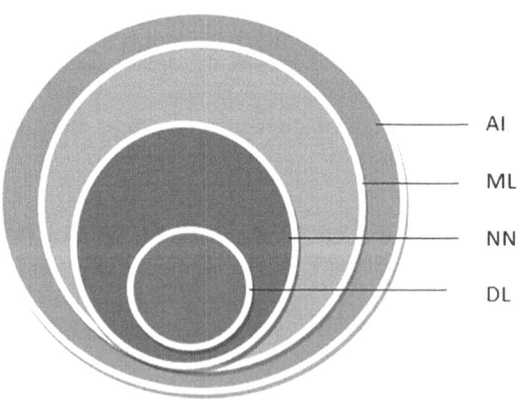

Fig. 1. Relationship between AI, ML, NN and DL

can monitor the patients and very good communication between doctors and patients. Figure 1. Shows the architecture of Neural network, Deep learning, Machine learning and AI.

5 Conclusion

Today big data have been used in different areas. One of these is mental healthcare system. Various smart devices have been used now a days for mental patients and by use of AI and sensor devices, the rate of death of mental patients reduced tremendously. We also surveyed about different models of ML algorithms to predict the mental patients. Naïve bayes, SVM, k-means and random forest have been commonly used to predict mental patients. Sentiment analysis can also be used for mental health prediction using data analytics on the social media. In future, with improving the accuracy, our aim of the work will give a better diagnosis of mental patients and using the twitter data, we can detect the depression for target patients using low cost-effective way.

References

1. Khattak, A., et al.: Data analytics in mental healthcare. Sci. Program. (2020)
2. Bauer, R., Glenn, T., Strejilevich, S., et al.: Internet use by older adults with bipolar disorder: international survey results. Int. J. Bipolar Disord. **6**(1), 20 (2018)
3. de Montjoye, Y.A., Quoidbach, J., Robic, F., Pentland, A.: Predicting personality using novel mobile phone-based metrics. In: Greenberg, A.M., Kennedy, W.G., Bos, N.D. (eds.) Social Computing, Behavioral-Cultural Modeling and Prediction. SBP 2013. Lecture Notes in Computer Science, vol. 7812, pp. 48–55. Springer, Berlin (2013). https://doi.org/10.1007/978-3-642-37210-0_6
4. Bauer, W., Hopwood, C.J.: Using machine learning to advance personality assessment and theory. Pers. Soc. Psychol. Rev. **23**(2), 190–203 (2019)
5. Hill, C., Martin, J.L., Thomson, S., Scott-Ram, N., Penfold, H., Creswell, C.: Navigating the challenges of digital health innovation: considerations and solutions in developing online and smartphone-application-based interventions for mental health disorders. Br. J. Psychiatry **211**(2), 65–69 (2017)
6. Dimitrov, D.V.: Medical internet of things and big data in healthcare. Healthc. Inf. Res. **22**(3), 156–163 (2016)
7. Monteith, S., Glenn, T., Geddes, J., Bauer, M.: Big data are coming to psychiatry: a general introduction. Int. J. Bipolar Disord. **3**(1), 21 (2015)
8. Kellmeyer, P.: Big brain data: on the responsible use of brain data from clinical and consumer-directed neuro technological devices. Neuroethics **11**, 1–16 (2018)
9. Jiang, L., Gao, B., Gu, J., et al.: Wearable long-term social sensing for mental wellbeing. IEEE Sens. J. **19**(19) (2019)
10. Yang, S., Gao, B., Jiang, L., et al.: IoT structured long-term wearable social sensing for mental wellbeing. IEEE Internet Things J. **6**(2), 3652–3662 (2018)
11. Monteith, S., Glenn, T.: Automated decision-making and big data: concerns for people with mental illness. Curr. Psychiatry Rep. **18**(12), 112 (2016)
12. Goyal, S.: Sentimental analysis of twitter data using text mining and hybrid classification approach. Int. J. Adv. Res. Ideas Innovations Technol. **2**(5), 2454–3132 (2016)

13. Kumar, M., Bala, A.: Analyzing twitter sentiments through big data. In: Proceedings of the 2016 3rd International Conference on Computing for Sustainable Global Development (INDIACom), pp. 2628–2631, New Delhi, India (2016)
14. Dhaka, P., Johari, R.: Big data application: study and archival of mental health data, using MongoDB. In: Proceedings of the 2016 International Conference on Electrical, Electronics, and Optimization Techniques (ICEEOT), pp. 3228–3232, Chennai, India (2016)
15. De Beurs, D., Van Bruinessen, I., Noordman, J., Friele, R., Van Dulmen, S.: Active involvement of end users when developing web-based mental health interventions. Front. Psych. **8**, 72 (2017)
16. Turner, V., Gantz, J.F., Reinsel, D., Minton, S.: e digital universe of opportunities: rich data and the increasing value of the internet of things. IDC Anal. Future **16** (2014)
17. Passos, I.C., Ballester, P., Pinto, J.V., Mwangi, B., Kapczinski, F.: Big data and machine learning meet the health sciences. In: Personalized Psychiatry, pp. 1–13. Springer, Cham, Switzerland (2019)
18. Kessler, R.C., Bernecker, S.L., Bossarte, R.M., et al.: e role of big data analytics in predicting suicide. In: Personalized Psychiatry, pp. 77–98, Springer, Cham, Switzerland (2019)
19. Cleland, B., Wallace, J., Bond, R., et al.: Insights into antidepressant prescribing using open health data. Big Data Res. **12**, 41–48 (2018)
20. Hasan, M.M., Patel, M.R., Modestino, A.S., Sanchez, L.D., Young, G.: A novel big data analytics framework to predict the risk of opioid use disorder (2019)
21. Perdue, R.T., Hawdon, J., Thames, K.M.: Can big data predict the rise of novel drug abuse?. J. Drug Issues **48**(4), 508–518 (2018)
22. Furnham, A.: A big five facet analysis of sub-clinical dependent personality disorder (dutifulness). Psychiatry Res. **270**, 622–626 (2018)
23. Salagre, E., Vieta, E., Grande, I.: Personalized treatment in bipolar disorder. In: Personalized Psychiatry, pp. 423–436, Academic Press, Cambridge, MA, USA (2020)
24. Granka, L.: Inferring the public agenda from implicit query data. In: Proceedings of the 32nd International ACM SIGIR Conference on Research and Development in Information Retrieval, Boston, MA, USA (2009)
25. Sinha, V.: (2019). https://www.quora.com/What-are-the-maindifferences-between-artificial-intelligence-and-machine-learningIs-machine-learning-a-part-of-artificial-intelligence
26. Lenhart, A., Purcell, K., Smith, A., Zickuhr, K.: Social media & mobile internet use among teens and young adults. Millennials. Pew Internet Am. Life Proj. Washington, DC, USA (2010)
27. de la Torre Díez, I., Alonso, S.G., Hamrioui, S., Cruz, E.M., Nozaleda, L.M., Franco, M.A.: IoT-based services and applications for mental health in the literature. J. Med. Syst. **43**(1), 11. PMID: 30519972 (2018). https://doi.org/10.1007/s10916-018-1130-3
28. Berdahl, C.H.: A neural network model of borderline personality disorder. Neural Netw. **23**(2), 177–188 (2010). https://doi.org/10.1016/j.neunet.2009.10.007. Epub 2009 Nov 10 PMID: 19932003

Author Index

A
Agrawal, Deepak 45

B
Barik, Shekharesh 21
Behera, Chandan Kumar 21
Behera, Pravat Kumar 21
Brahmachary, Subhranshu Nanda 21

D
Dwivedi, Anjana 1

K
Kayal, Mrinmoy 72
Khate, Kevisino 12
Kondaveeti, Hari Kishan 59
Kumar, Basant 45

N
Neelima, Arambam 12, 33

P
Pati, Jayadeep 72

S
Sahoo, Mohinikanta 72
Sarmah, Mriganka 33
Sarmah, Puspakshi 33
Satapathy, Santosh Kumar 59
Shah, Vaishvi R. 59
Sharma, Gaurav 45
Singh, Aakansha 1
Singh, Maninder 45
Soni, K. M. 45

The manufacturer's authorised representative in the EU is Springer Nature Customer Service Centre GmbH, Europaplatz 3, 69115 Heidelberg, Germany. If you have any concerns regarding our products, please contact ProductSafety@springernature.com

Printed and bound by CPI Group (UK) Ltd, Croydon, CR0 4YY

26/03/2026

02078935-0015